MOON PATH YOGA

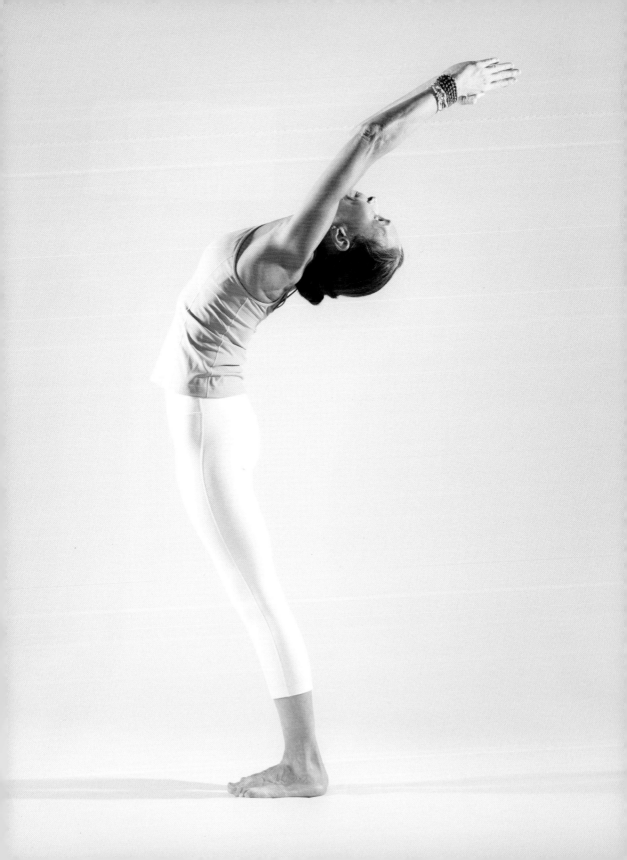

MOON PATH YOGA

Kundalini Practices and Rituals for Women
to Align with the Lunar Cycles

SIERRA HOLLISTER

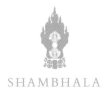

SHAMBHALA

Shambhala Publications, Inc.
2129 13th Street
Boulder, Colorado 80302
www.shambhala.com

Cover art: Artsem Vysotski/VikaSuh/Shutterstock.com
Cover and interior design: Laura Shaw Design

9 8 7 6 5 4 3 2 1

FIRST EDITION
Printed in China

Shambhala Publications makes every effort
to print on acid-free, recycled paper.
Shambhala Publications is distributed worldwide by
Penguin Random House, Inc., and its subsidiaries.

LIBRARY OF CONGRESS CATALOGING-IN-PUBLICATION DATA

Names: Hollister, Sierra, author.
Title: Moon path yoga: Kundalini practices and rituals for women to
align with the lunar cycles / Sierra Hollister.
Description: Boulder: Shambhala, 2022.
Identifiers: LCCN 2021049450 | ISBN 9781611809558 (trade paperback)
Subjects: LCSH: Kuṇḍalinī. | Moon—Phases. | Yoga—Therapeutic use. | Women and religion.
Classification: LCC BL1238.56.K86 H65 2022 | DDC 294.5/436—dc23/eng/20211117
LC record available at https://lccn.loc.gov/2021049450

This book is dedicated to the
many beautiful souls—students, teachers, and
colleagues—who have shared the practice of yoga
with me over the past three decades. Yoga is a path
that seeks to deliver us to our wisest, kindest selves.
The sincere practice of yoga offers a lifetime of learning,
timeless guidance on conduct and life, and infinite
opportunities to experience love, challenge, humility,
expansion, and connection. In recognition of the way
we shape each other in relationship, always
creating our future selves with each interaction,
this book belongs to you.

Thank you.

CONTENTS

Practice List

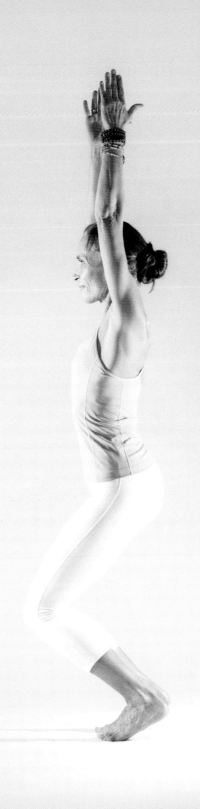

Introduction

IT IS ABSOLUTELY thrilling to me that you are holding this book in your hands! My deepest wish is that this book becomes a valuable touchstone for you, one that you turn to again and again. When I picture this book living in your home, I imagine it worn and tattered through continual use, stained with rings from your tea (or coffee!) cup, and filled with dog-eared pages galore. Perhaps it will even have some flowers pressed within its pages or feathers marking your place. These are the visual cues that a book has earned status and become a cherished source. More than anything else, this book is a guide to walking the path illuminated by the moon, a path that will take you into deeper self-knowing.

The Moon Path is the path that all who identify as women walk, whether they realize it or not. The Moon Path is the path of life, of light, of dark. To realize the Moon Path is to awaken to your deepest knowing of yourself as a lunar being. On this path, we attune to the way the moon is with us in all that we do. For some of us that will include the moon being with us in bleeding and birthing; for others, the relationship with the moon will call in other ways. For all of us, the moon is experienced from sleeping to waking, from cradle to grave. Various cultures over time have positioned the moon in relationship as Mother or Grandmother, as Sister or Goddess. It is for you to determine if the moon is your beloved sister or unconditionally loving mother, your wise grandmother or goddess energy to invoke. Or it may be that the moon sings for you in a fluid, nonbinary voice and you summon in the same. No matter how you relate to the moon, know this for certain: she was with you before you were born, when you were just a whisper in the womb, and she will carry you through this life, always.

Let these teachings hold you as they have held women through time. Share these teachings with other women, other sisters. Share these teachings with anyone and everyone whom you feel called to, as those who resonate with moon energy can identify anywhere along the gender spectrum, from nonbinary to binary. These teachings are not exclusive and to share them is to open the circle of moon. In this way, you are part of the silver and golden chain of carrying these ways forward, ensuring their survival.

May you thrive in the light of the moon; may you find rest in her dark. May you realize a global sisterhood and use some of your beautiful energy on behalf of that sisterhood. So long as one suffers, none are liberated—and yoga is a call to liberation and wholeness for all.

MOON PATH YOGA

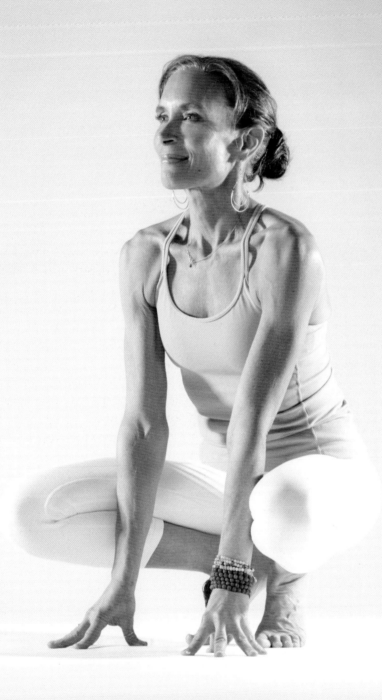

1

Walking the Moon Path

THIS BOOK IS like the moon path itself—circular, from new to full and back again. Open to any section that calls you. Read, practice, meditate. With the exception of contraindications for bleeding times and pregnancy, all the sequences can be practiced whenever you want, as often as you want. If you are bleeding or pregnant, please read the chapters "Practices for Moon Times" and "We Are All Mothers" before practicing other sequences. You'll want to familiarize yourself with how we care for our bodies during those times. Once you understand those suggestions, you can modify other sequences for practice during times of bleeding (moon time) and pregnancy.

Over the years of teaching, I've had numerous women ask if these practices will still be beneficial if they have had a hysterectomy. A hysterectomy is a surgical procedure to remove the uterus and can range from a subtotal hysterectomy (removal of the main body of the uterus, leaving cervix in place) to a radical hysterectomy (uterus, fallopian tubes, ovaries, lymph glands, and portions of the vagina are removed) with options in between. The answer to the question is a resounding yes! Even though there is organ removal, the energetic channels and functions remain. The practice of yoga, especially kundalini yoga, is predicated upon the subtle body anatomy illuminated by the ancient seers. This anatomy is about energetic pathways, energy fields and bodies, and of course, the way that prana, or life force, moves through your body. So while Western anatomy is incumbent upon the visible—organs and muscles and physical structure—subtle body anatomy is about the invisible, the flow of energy. Although you might live in a body that no longer has ovaries—or a spleen or tonsils or another organ, for that matter—the energetic meridians of that organ are still intact. Vitality and energy are still flowing through those pathways. We are still able to step into the power and beauty of yoga practice and nourish ourselves in very

The word *kriya* is Sanskrit for "action" and implies that the action is complete, a blossoming. Sometimes the words *kriya* and *sequence* are used interchangeably, yet (in contrast to a kriya) a sequence might not be fully complete in its action. In kundalini yoga, the word *kriya* is most often used when referring to a sequence of actions, because the distinct practices of this tradition are considered whole and entire in impact and integration.

deep ways, regardless of the details of our personal physical structure because we are tapping into a mystical and universal energetic structure.

Within us, a magical universe exists, and outside of us, the numinous beckons. When we open our eyes to the sheer wonder of the earth, the allure and enchantments held in the sky above us, we are affirming what has thrummed in our spirit all along. In this way, we approach the moon, ready to decode what has been whispered to us from the sky for our entire lives.

One of the many ways that we can deepen our relationship to the moon, as well as our relationship to the natural world, is by journaling. As you explore the Moon Path, your journal can be enhanced by collecting information that tracks your unique relationship with the moon. Chapter 3 includes a reproducible chart on page 37 that gives you a place to make notes about the times, places, and ways in which the moon lands in your body, along with room for noting your bleeding cycle and recording what phase the moon was in. You may find this chart helpful for identifying the movement of the moon through your body. You can make as many copies as needed of this chart: make twelve copies and track through the year, year in and year out, or make just a few copies and use it simply to establish your cycles. Feel free to use it, or not use it, in whatever way fits into the rhythm of your life with ease.

The numerous sequences, meditations, and mantras contained within this book originate primarily from the kundalini yoga lineage. Written descriptions of kundalini yoga date back to the Upanishadic era, approximately the fifth century B.C.E., and the oral tradition is, of course, much older. Deeply rooted in tantric philosophy, the kundalini yogic path is structured to awaken and is often referred to as "the yoga of awareness." Each of us is a divine and unique expression of nature and life force and each of us lives in a body that expresses our uniqueness in different ways, on different days. Some days, I enjoy a leisurely and slow warm-up for my body before entering a *kriya* (sequence). (See sidebar.) Other days, I find that I want to jump right into a practice or meditation, with no preliminaries. As long as you honor yourself and what is real for you when it comes to your practice (and life)—there is no wrong way.

TIPS, TOOLS, AND ILLUMINATIONS

As you work your way through this book, you might encounter various terms or techniques that are new to you or are expressed differently than in other yogic traditions. The explanatory section below offers a full illumination of the tools and techniques specifically utilized in this book.

MANTRAS

Mantra, like yoga, is science, art, technology, and sacred. Numerous ways and numerous traditions teach that "at the beginning" was the word, or sound. Mantra is sacred sound, encoded with vibratory frequencies that find resonance in the universe and invoke precise patterns and motions. Mantra works with the coding of the universe as well as the coding of the individual. When we chant, our tongue strikes various meridian points in the mouth; in this way, the chant also elicits corresponding effects on the various organ and glandular systems related to the meridian points. I believe that mantra is best chanted with reverence and gratitude, while humbly remembering that access to mantra is a profound gift. Described below are various mantras you will encounter in this book.

ONG NAMO, GURU DEV NAMO. This mantra translates as "I bow to the subtle divine wisdom, I bow to the teacher in my heart" and is known as the *adi* mantra. *Adi* means "first" or "primary," and the adi mantra is the invocation used most often to begin the practice of kundalini. If you chant this mantra as an invocation before each practice, you are acknowledging the wisdom that pervades the universe and also remembering and affirming the teacher residing within; the invocation serves as a way to open to all that is possible and at the same time draw a boundary of protection and integrity. Over time, the vibration of the mantra sings in your body and unlocks subtle knowing as well as healing. (If this particular mantra doesn't resonate for you, however, I encourage you to seek out a mantra that does.)

INVOCATION WITH MANTRA

At the start of your practice, seated or standing, before engaging with your chosen mantra, consider bringing your hands together at your heart and gently rubbing them, creating a gentle warming with the friction. This brings the Shakti of the heart forward. *Shakti* means "power" or "energy," but it especially suggests the divine feminine creative aspect of power. Allow a few breaths to simply notice any sensation or feeling that is generated with this action. Most often, a warming and opening sensation blossoms at the heart, but there can be other sensations too—anticipation, curiosity, joy, and more. You can sing your chosen mantra, speak it, or simply think it. Three repetitions of the mantra are said to cover the past, the present, and the future. Over time, the recitation of the mantra becomes entwined with the pleasure of practicing; eventually, as you recite your mantra, your body feels that pleasure in the recitation.

WAHE GURU. The connotation of this mantra points to the bliss, or ecstasy beyond words, of moving "from the darkness of ignorance to the light of knowing." This mantra is sweet, simple, and so affirming.

GURU GURU WAHE GURU, GURU RAM DAS GURU. This mantra is profoundly healing and lends itself to a number of different rhythms and melodies. It is often referred to as the "miracle mantra." GURU is one who takes you from the dark to the light, a teacher. WAHE is bliss—or more accurately, ecstasy that defies words. RAM DAS was the fourth guru of the ten Gurus of Sikhism, the creators and sustainers of the Sikh religion over a period of approximately two hundred years. Guru Ram Das was noted for his service, the power of his presence, and his seemingly infinite and open heart. It was said that miracles of healing happened in his attendance. When we chant this mantra, we invoke the energy of the heart, of miracles, and of self-healing. You do not need to be Sikh—or any religion—to invoke this energy in your practice.

SAT NAM. This mantra is considered to be a *bija*, or "seed," mantra. Seed mantras are short and incredibly powerful; like a seed, they contain everything for growth and manifestation. SAT means "true" or "truth," and NAM means "self" or "identity." To chant SAT NAM is to affirm and strengthen your truest self.

SA TA NA MA. This mantra is known as the *panj shabd* and represents the ever-spinning wheel of creation. SA means "infinity," TA means "life," NA means "death" or "transformation," and MA stands for "birth" or "rebirth." In yogic thought, our soul is always somewhere on this wheel, infinitely cycling through the never-ending wheel of existence.

MA. In the *panj shabd*, this syllable represents birth or rebirth. Alone, as sound current, MA also stands for both "moon" and "mother."

PRANAYAMA

Prana, a component of our breath, is life, and the yogic tradition includes hundreds of ways to work with your breath, in practices called *pranayama*. The pranayama techniques you will use in this book are described below. If no instructions for the breath are given in a particular sequence you encounter later in this book, allow an organic, natural breath while you do the practice—a breath that is not exaggerated but that may be a little fuller than you tend to breathe without noticing.

NATURAL BREATH. Breathe with a relaxed belly and relaxed yet lifted diaphragm. Take between 5 and 7 seconds for the inhale; the exhale should match in duration. Allow the belly to soften and gently expand with the inhale and contract with the exhale.

LONG DEEP BREATHING. This is a conscious expansion and lengthening of the natural breath. It could be 8–12 seconds on the inhale, matching the exhale in duration. A long deep breath has more expansion as well as contraction in movement, and the top as well as bottom of the breath will also be felt in the top of the chest by the collarbones.

BREATH OF FIRE (*agni pran*). This pranayama is achieved by pumping your navel and connecting the breath. When you pull the navel in, your breath is expelled—usually through the nose but, depending on the kriya, it could be through the mouth. By actively pulling the navel in, the breath is activated by the exhale. As the navel releases, the inhale happens and is calibrated to match the exhale. Breath of fire can be gentle or powerful, depending upon the sequence.

ALTERNATE NOSTRIL BREATHING (*nadi shodhan*). Numerous variations of this pranayama utilize the left and the right nostril in different ways. All alternate nostril breathing is working with the *ida nadi* (left nostril, moon energy) and the *pingala nadi* (right nostril, sun energy) for specific outcomes. Utilizing the left nostril is soothing, cooling, and calming. Utilizing the right nostril is activating, warming, and clarifying. Working in various combinations with both of these nadis, by working with both nostrils, creates balance.

SEGMENTED BREATHING. This pranayama breaks our inhale and our exhale into different "segments." Each of the segmented breath practices brings known and reliable effects. Two different segments are suggested in this book: one uses a 4:1 (inhale in four equal sniffs or segments and exhale in one unbroken segment); the other is 4:8 (inhale in four equal segments and exhale in eight equal segments).

SITALI PRANAYAMA. This breathing technique is extraordinary and powerful. In *sitali* breathing ("breathing through the beak"), the practitioner rolls the tongue into a U shape and puts the tongue out, inhaling through and over the curled tongue. The most traditional variation has the practitioner then draw the tongue back into the mouth, close the mouth, and exhale slowly through the nose. The effects are noticeably cooling and calming as well as elevating. I encourage readers to try this way of breathing and note the effects for themselves, adding it to your personal inventory of practices that are soothing. In chapter 7, a version of sitali pranayama, stylized with breath of fire energy is used.

CANNON BREATH. Most often, and in this book, cannon breath is a powerful exhale through the mouth—as if you were releasing a cannon.

MUDRA

The word *mudra* can mean a number of different things depending upon context as well as the location of the person using the term. The word itself means "sacred gesture" or "seal" and can refer to the positioning of the hands, the eyes, the body, and even the breath. In this book, *mudra* will always refer to a position the hands take. Mudras are used all over the world, in many different cultures. The source of the mudras that I share in *Moon Path Yoga* originate primarily from the Punjabi region of India with one exception: *Anjali* mudra, which seems to be universal in form, although differing in name. My understanding of the mudras that I share is sourced from kundalini, tantra, and hatha teachings.

Mudras can be linked to the energy of the consciousness, the flow of subtle-body anatomy, planetary influences, deity energy, and more. What is always true is that our fingertips are dense with nerves that communicate with our brain constantly and efficiently; this communication flows below our conscious awareness.

GYAN MUDRA (the seal of knowledge). This mudra is formed by placing the tip of the thumb to the tip of the index finger (also known as the "Jupiter" finger). This seal is said to signal receptivity to receiving wisdom and knowledge. Taking this mudra can feel calming while also enhancing our receptivity.

SHUNI MUDRA (the seal of patience). This mudra is formed by placing the tip of the thumb to the tip of the middle finger (the "Saturn" finger); along with signaling a desire for patience, it creates a wavelength of discernment. This mudra can help us with commitment and responsibility.

SURYA MUDRA (the seal of the sun). This mudra is formed by placing the tip of the third finger to the tip of the thumb, beckoning vitality and health and strengthening the nervous system.

BUDDHI MUDRA (the seal of mental clarity and communication). Created by touching the thumb tip to the tip of the fourth finger (the "Mercury" finger), this mudra signals the desire for higher understanding, intuitive knowing, and clear communication.

VENUS MUDRA (named for the Venus mound, the ample area of the palm below the thumb). This mudra is formed by interlacing the fingers of both hands together. Sealing our hands in the Venus mudra is said to channel our sexual and creative energy in a way that allows us to focus. This mudra is also thought to be beneficial to our glandular system.

ANJALI MUDRA (also known as *pranam* mudra, or the Prayer Pose, a globally sacred gesture). The palms come together at the heart; uniting moon (left hand/side of the body) and sun (right hand/side of the body). This seal can represent many things; it is used in expressing petitions, wishes, prayers, gratitude for divine gifts, reverent and respectful greetings, or an open and engaged heart.

The mudras in this book can be likened to *asanas* (yogic postures) for the hands. In some kriyas in the following pages, the hands are positioned in a specific way that is not a traditional mudra, to create the opportunity to enhance the flow of energy in a way that is explicit to that sequence. Our entire hand, but especially the thumb and fingers, is connected not only to the elements but also to certain planetary energies, from a Vedic viewpoint.

The thumb has no planetary association, instead representing the individual ego as well as the ability to transcend the ego and experience universal consciousness. The thumb is associated with the element of fire. The index finger corresponds to the planet Jupiter; it has the energy of expansiveness, big and abundant. The element associated with the index finger is air, also expansive. The middle finger is linked to Saturn, an energy that is thought to be demanding, exacting—a "task-master," so to speak—and the element is ether (sometimes referred to as space). The third finger (the "ring finger") brings the energy of the sun, life-giving and vital. Here we draw courage and find consistency. Earth is the element linked to the third finger. The fourth finger (or "little finger") signifies Mercury—motion, quickness, the linking power of communication. Water is the element of the fourth finger.

BANDHAS

Bandha is a Sanskrit word meaning "lock" or "close off." In yoga, bandhas are a way of working with, or locking, the channels (nadis) in which prana flows through the body—that is, by engaging specific muscles and employing specific techniques, the practitioner is able to create internal locks to work with energy flows in the body. Four primary bandhas are utilized in kundalini practices.

JALANDHAR **BANDHA.** Although this technique is often referred to as the "neck lock" or "chin lock," that rendering is a bit of a misnomer. A more accurate translation might be "locking the throat stream." Jalandhar bandha is perhaps the most frequently employed lock, done primarily in a seated position. To work this lock, sit tall with the chest lifted. Lengthen your neck by subtly drawing the chin straight back (not down). Your throat should be barely engaged; the lock should be a consequence of drawing the chin back, not of effort. Jalandhar bandha works with energy in the upper body; it can be done on the inhale or the exhale and is often held during meditation and or chanting.

MULA **BANDHA.** This bandha, the "root lock," can be done on the inhale or the exhale in any number of positions and actions. To engage this lock, the rectum is contracted, the sexual organs are lifted within the body, and the navel point is drawn back toward the spine. This lock is said to blend and balance the two primary pranic winds in the body (prana exists as *maha prana*, or great prana, throughout the universe. This maha prana is within us as well and depending on where the prana is dwelling, takes on certain characteristics and attributes. Mula bandha blends apana and prana. For more on the five winds of prana within us, refer to page 41. Mula bandha also stimulates the flow of spinal fluid and opens the main channel for kundalini energy to rise. (Note: this lock is contraindicated while menstruating. For more information, refer to the chapter "Practices for Moon Times.")

UDDIYANA BANDHA. Also known as the "diaphragm lock," this bandha is only engaged with the breath out. To engage uddiyana bandha, exhale completely and with the lungs empty, suspend breathing while pulling the entire abdominal region both up under the ribs and back toward the spine. Your chest and sternum should be lifted and your lower spine softly brought forward. To release the lock, relax the abdomen and slowly inhale. This lock massages the internal organs, brings energy to the heart, and is thought to integrate the emotional and the physical.

MAHA BANDHA. This is the "great lock," when all three primary bandhas are engaged at the same time—consequently, this lock is always done only on the exhale. Maha bandha is believed to work with the entire subtle body anatomy and initiate healing where needed.

DHRISTI

Dhristi is the focus of our gaze, and this word's translation from Sanskrit is "gaze" or "vision" or "concentrated sight." Dhristi refers to ways in which we can focus our eyes as we practice. Generally, in kundalini, if no specific dhristi is mentioned, we close our eyes and allow ourselves to go inward. Some of the practices in this book will direct your eyes to the brow point (or "third eye"). Sometimes the gaze is lifted to the crown of the head, as if you could look through and see the sky. Other times, the gaze is downward, to the chin, the heart, or the floor. Fixing your gaze on the horizon or a steady spot on the floor can be helpful during balancing postures.

Teachings from the Yoga Sutras mention that energy (prana) follows attention (focus) and that we can harness this principle by consciously fixing our focus. This is true in our actual practice of yoga but also as we live our practice out in the world. This attention to focus can shape our larger view of the world, and shape the flow of energy to that view and the action we take. To some extent, embarking on the Moon Path and awakening to the power and the influence of the moon is a dhristi, a compass of sorts. Consciously considering and directing our dhristi is a way of cultivating wisdom and insight as well as a way to shape our relationship to the world.

PREPARING TO PRACTICE

As emphasized earlier, there are no rules here; what follows is simply an invitation to the lunar path and its practices with the hope that these teachings will provide sustenance, harmony, and meaning. Over the course of thirty years of practice, I have found great value in warming my physical body up with movement as a means of preparing myself for practicing the kriyas. With that said, I know many practitioners who simply jump right into the kriyas with no priming.

Should you wish to warm up before practicing one of the sequences or meditations offered in the book, I am sharing two of my favorite ways to begin my practice. The first is a fairly traditional and simple way: the **Seated Warm-Up.** The second is a more flowing way to prepare your body for practice: the **Gentle Salutation**. There have been days when one or both of these two ways to warm up are actually my entire practice! I hope you enjoy the way these warm-up options feel. Another option is to simply allow your body to move intuitively on your mat, tuning in to your hips, the backs of your legs, your spine and shoulders. Your warm-up does not have to look a certain way, nor does it need to have a "proper" asana name to be of value.

SEATED WARM-UP

1. Take a simple cross-legged seat, a posture known as Sukhasana. Inhale, flexing your spine forward, chest lifted; then exhale, flexing your spine back. Allow a subtle forward motion on the bones of your seat as you inhale, backward motion as you exhale. Begin slowly, noticing your body, gradually increasing in speed if it feels right. Spinal flexes are an excellent way to prepare the spine for yoga. Continue for 2–3 minutes.

▷

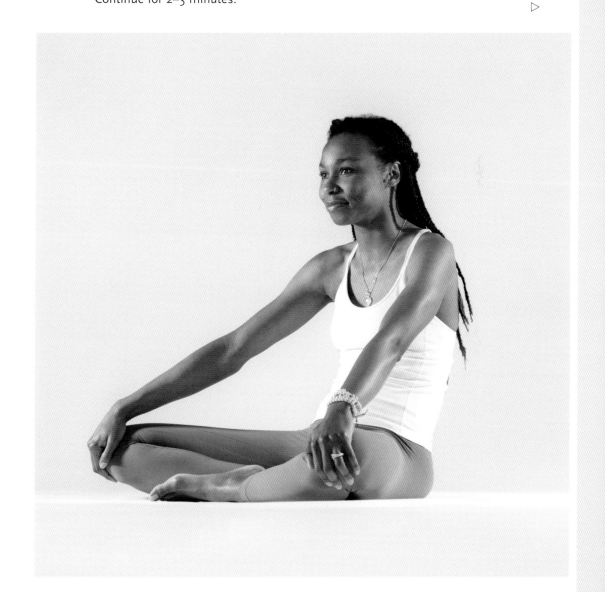

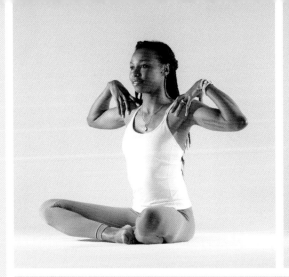
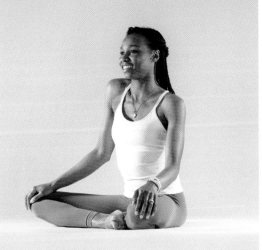
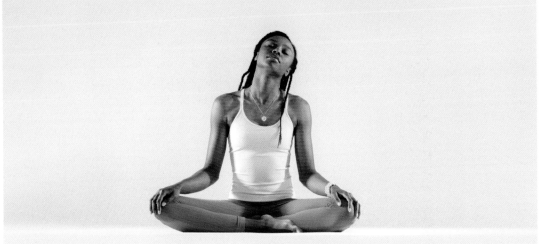

2. Still in Sukhasana, bring your hands to your shoulders, with fingertips to the front of your shoulders and thumbs behind. Inhale as you twist left; exhale as you twist right. Continue twisting at a comfortable pace for 1–2 minutes.

3. In the same seat, begin to alternately roll one shoulder at a time, moving blade and muscle. Take your time and allow yourself to feel gratitude for all the work that your shoulders do. Do this for 1–2 minutes.

4. Focus your thought on your neck as you lengthen it. For those who have sustained spinal cord injuries or cervical vertebrae injuries, slowly turn your head side to side, keeping your chin level. If you are injury-free, explore neck rolls by slowly circling your head in one direction 5–10 times. Return to the center, pausing a moment as you re-lengthen the neck, then continue circling an equal amount of times in the other direction.

5. This next series of movement consists of three different postures known collectively as the "life nerve stretch." In the kundalini tradition, the sciatic nerve is often referred to as the body's "life nerve," because the state of this nerve can greatly impact our quality of life.

» Unfold your legs straight out in front of you and bring your heels together. Flex your heels forward, bringing your toes back toward your torso. Lift your arms up over your head with your next inhale; on the exhale, fold forward. Relax the upper body, while still keeping the backs of your legs on the floor. It is more important to keep the backs of your legs to the floor than to grasp your toes, so resting your hands on your shins or knees is fine too. Breathe long and deep in this forward fold for 2 minutes.

» Release from the previous position, lifting your arms up over your head, inhaling as you rise. Relax and draw your left heel up toward your groin, with your left foot relaxed and touching your right inner thigh. Lift your arms with an inhale, then fold with the exhale. This posture is much like the last one, but here you are working with just one leg rather than both. Continue in this forward folded position, breathing for about 2 minutes. Then release upward with the inhale and switch legs, repeating on the other side.

» Spread your legs comfortably wide and flex your heels forward again. Inhale and lift your arms up over the head, with the torso centered. Exhale and fold forward over your left leg. Rise back to the center with the next inhale. Exhale and fold forward over your right leg. Continue moving with the breath, inhaling in the center and exhaling down to alternate sides, flowing for about 2 minutes.

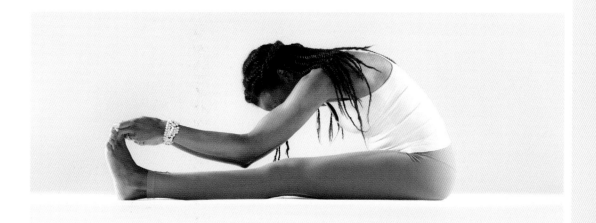

GENTLE SALUTATION

Allow as many repetitions for this practice as you need to feel limber and warm; 10–12 rounds can be lovely, but each body is unique. Sometimes I like to begin with the **Gentle Salutation** and then, after a few rounds, move on to another salutation.

1. Standing, come to the top of your mat and bring your hands into Anjali mudra at the heart. Feel into your feet, drawing up the energy of earth. Notice your posture and adjust accordingly to be tall yet relaxed.

2. Inhale, lifting your arms over your head.

3. Exhale, folding forward to the floor.

4. Inhale, halfway up, lifting the heart and head to the horizon.

5. Exhale, folding back down, fingertips to the earth as you send your left leg back.

6. Inhale as you lift and extend into Warrior 1 Pose (Virabhadrasana)

7. Exhale, bringing your fingertips forward as you switch your legs, bringing your left leg forward and sending your right leg back.

8. Inhale to Warrior 1 Pose (now on other side).

9. Exhale, with your fingers forward, drawing your back leg forward and bringing feet together.

10. Inhale, halfway up, lifting the heart and the head to the horizon.

11. Exhale, folding forward.

12. Inhale, lifting your arms over your head, stretching straight up.

13. Exhale, returning your hands to Anjali mudra at the heart.

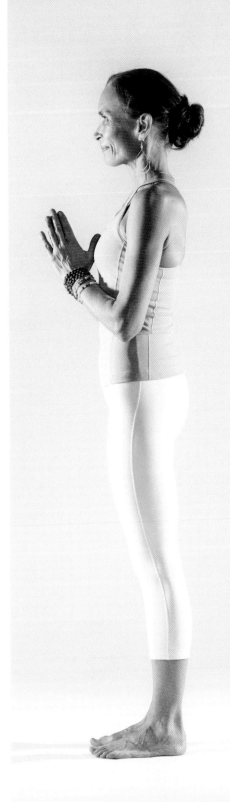

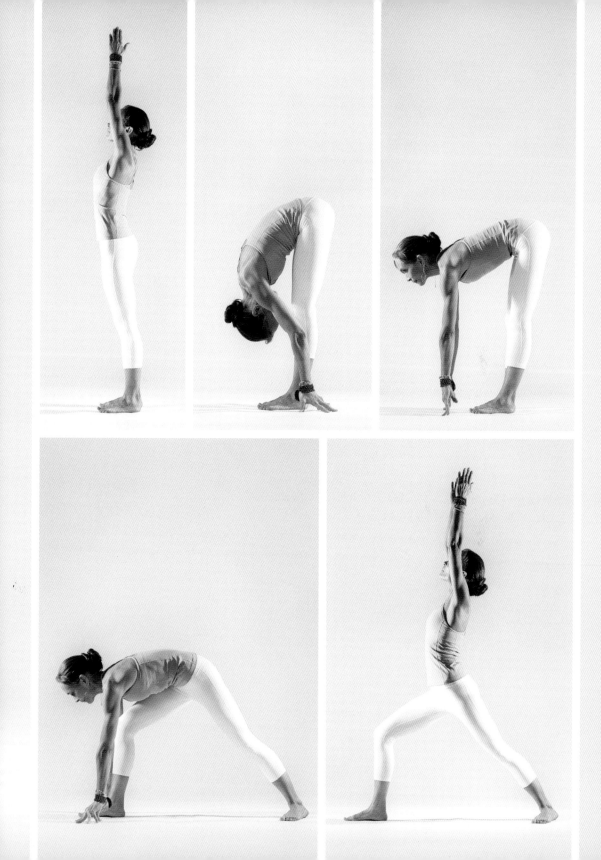

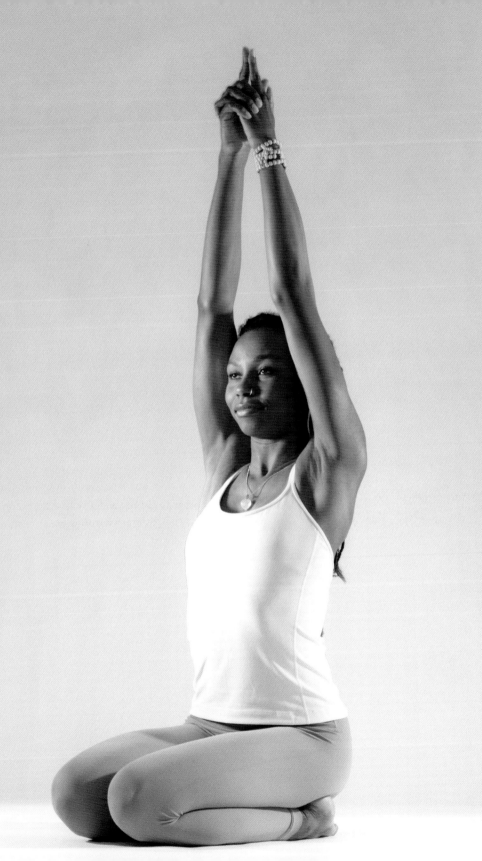

2

Woman Is a Lunar Being

YOU ARE HOLDING this book in your hands right now because at some level, you intuitively and deeply understand that you are in relationship with the moon and that this relationship is both mystical and practical, both somatically rooted and ephemerally compelling. This relationship to the moon, as one who identifies as woman, is significant.

In powerful ways, the moon speaks to all of us, from the moment of our conception to the last breath we draw. *La luna* stands out, surrounded by dark, casting illumination and guidance. She is cooling and calm, soothing and serene, and yet she can arouse us with her energy and force. She reflects the light of the sun and yet has the power to move the waters of the entire Earth. Not only does she impact the entire animal world with her presence or absence, but she also shapes behavior and ritual within species. The effect of the moon on plant life is well documented and the *Farmer's Almanac* has long included sections on planting and harvesting according to the phase of the moon.

Women have a deep, profound, and unique relationship with the moon. The moon moves through our bodies, in a cycle that was established while we were still in our mother's womb—this is our "moon center cycle." As well, our monthly bleeding is connected to the moon and her phases—this is our moon cycle. Just like the moon, we wax and fill and wane and empty. The moon influences the time and flow of our blood, and as you'll learn in the next chapter, she dances through our bodies in a pattern that impacts our moods, our behavior, and our choices.

THE TIMELESS POLARITIES OF STABLE AND FLOW

Woman has been associated with the moon since far back in ancient history—as demonstrated in the nature of goddess-based religions and by the mythology, ritual, and other aspects of countless cultures and traditions that identify the moon as feminine. In contrast, the sun has come to represent the masculine in many wisdom traditions and healing paths. But crucially, men feel the moon as well, and women, of course, are influenced by the sun. Ayurveda (one of the world's oldest healing traditions and, like yoga, sourced from the Vedas) recognizes that a primary requirement for well-being, for all of us, is harmonizing our cycles with the larger cycles of the moon, sun, and Earth. In this light, and regardless of how you identify, to consider the moon as strictly feminine and the sun as strictly masculine is to ignore the reality that gender is a spectrum as well as a social construct—and to consider gender as simply binary is to miss the beauty and diversity of all that surrounds us, has come before us, and is still to come. It is true that we can acknowledge that all of us are impacted by the moon, sun, and Earth while also honoring that those who identify as women have a special affinity for the moon, a deeper relationship with the cycles and phases of the moon.

The soul itself is without gender, and the ancient yogic teachings maintain that we incarnate between Earth and the ethers in order to have particular experiences. Our soul chooses to incarnate in the body that it does to learn specific lessons and have specific experiences. These lessons and experiences bring us closer to wholeness and wisdom and are the tools that our soul uses to evolve.

At the heart of the ancient and timeless teachings of yoga is the understanding of polarity and the interrelationship and balance of opposites. The principle of polarity is manifest across the universe as well as within us. All of us, regardless of gender identification, contain lunar and solar energies. Our yogic ancestors discovered and charted an anatomy that is invisible to the eye and understood more readily with our consciousness than a microscope. This system of anatomy is referenced as the subtle body. The subtle body holds the fields and structures of energy flow, including the nadis, the channels through which prana flows. Of the many nadis, three are considered primary: *sushumna*, *ida*, and *pingala*. The sushumna runs up the spine to the crown of the head and is the route of the rising kundalini. The ida is our moon channel, originating at the base of the spine, to the left of the sushumna. The pingala is our sun channel, beginning at the base of the spine, to the right of the sushumna. The moon and sun channels crisscross the sushumna, weaving upward like a double helix and then ending at our nostrils—moon at the left nostril, sun at the right. Subtle body anatomy illustrates that we all embody both moon and sun, both flow and stable polarities. Our flow polarity is fluid, waning and waxing, filling and emptying. Flow rules our emotions and feelings, our connection to nature and the sensual, our experience of the moment. Flow can sometimes be clear and bright, sometimes submerged and mysterious. As you learn to identify this aspect of yourself, consider the moon and how she moves for clues. Our stable polarity is fixed, committed, an anchor; the stable features of our self rule our consciousness, our intellect, our ability to honor our commitments, and our long-term plans and visions. Stable is like the sun, consistent and visible. To identify this part of yourself, consider the sun and the way he moves.

As far as identifications such as male or female, the kundalini teachings (based on and sourced from the tantric teachings) are clear. Our identification as female or male is simply based on which polarity is strongest or even simply incrementally larger within us. It has nothing to do with our genitalia and everything to do with flow polarity and stable polarity. The flow polarity is moon ruled and holds the characteristics we've come to associate with the feminine. The stable polarity is ruled by the sun and is associated with masculine characteristics.

Western culture tends to refer to qualities of polarity as masculine and feminine, rather than solar and lunar, or stable and flow. In the tantric tradition, however, every aspect of the universe arises from a sacred source, and that includes us, regardless of the nomenclature we choose.

To identify as a woman is to be flow dominant, to be ruled by the moon. Women are lunar beings. Many of us know this intuitively as a result of our bleeding cycles. Our ovulation tends to sync with the moon cycle and we feel the pull of the moon as keenly as the tides. For many women our reproductive organs, our ages, and our changing relationship to our ovaries help define our life's stages and passages—but being a lunar being most certainly does not require ovaries. If you identify as a woman, then you are a lunar being.

As the natural world is cycling, women are connected to this cycle and going through our own cycles. Our ancient maternal ancestors noted the correlations and connections between the cycles of earth and sky, ovulation and bleeding, the orbital path of the moon, and created the system of charting the moon centers in this book. I would imagine, from the very first issue of menstrual blood, somewhere on the African continent, women have been tracking their bleeding, their moon time. Somewhere along the line, wise and intuitive maternal ancestors also began to correlate the movements of the moon somatically throughout the body, a rhythmic pattern that you will discover for yourself, known as the "moon center cycle."

As lunar beings, we embody the qualities of the moon—filling and emptying, being both luminescent and dark, exerting our own push and pull. One of my earliest kundalini yoga teachers often said that women take fourteen days to wax and fourteen days to wane, in the completion of the average twenty-eight-day moon cycle. To connect ourselves more consciously with the moon is a way of remembering our place in nature more fully.

Walking the Moon Path consciously, with care and attention, is one of the greatest gifts you can give to yourself; it will continue to nourish you in body, mind, and spirit through the years. Understanding the larger cycles of sun, moon, and Earth will enhance your ability to be in rhythm with nature and ultimately that understanding is crucial to your health and well-being. On the Moon Path, you will connect not only to your deepest, truest self but also to your maternal ancestors through time and ultimately to the divine feminine that pervades the universe and offers equilibrium to humanity—a healing counterweight to a world long imbalanced and biased to the masculine.

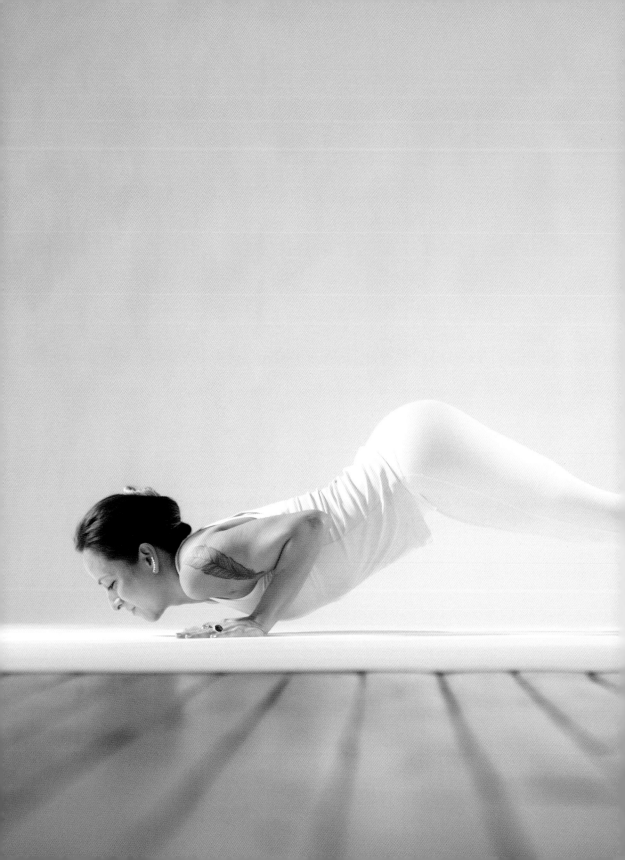

3

Charting Moon Cycles and Phases

HREE CYCLES ARE central to consider in deepening your intimacy with the moon. One cycle that you will need to learn, observe, and know about is the moon's own cycle, her orbital journey, which we'll look at later in this chapter. The other two of the three cycles happen within us, and the first of those, which we'll look at right now, is the bleeding cycle.

YOUR BODY MOVES WITH THE MOON: THE BLEEDING CYCLE

The moon interacts with our bodies in many ways, one of which can be monthly bleeding. Not all who identify as women have a bleeding cycle and not everyone who bleeds identifies as a woman. For those of us who do bleed, this cycle will not be with us for our entire lives. Still, the association of the monthly blood and the moon has been known, no doubt, since the first women bled. Our monthly blood has many, many names—shaped by geography and culture. Unfortunately, in many parts of the world, patriarchal fear (and lack of understanding) has defined women's monthly blood as something that is dirty, impure, and even dangerous. This has led to shame and taboo around what is essentially a beautiful gift, a gift that not only has the potential to create new life but also anchors us deeply to earth and the larger natural world, including the moon.

Some of the present-day euphemisms for monthly bleeding reflect cloaking, secrecy, and ambivalence. Mainstream cultural references to this cycle range from the subtle to the violent: among the literally thousands of different codes that have been used for this cycle—depending on where as well as when—we have "that time," "girlfriend," "the visit," "moon time" (various Indigenous people of North America), "little sister has come" (Chinese), "strawberry week" (German), "on the rag," "red tide," "shark week," "the curse." I came of bleeding age in the early eighties and at that time, in the culture I was reared, the term was *period*. I was told that I "had my period" and that was how I referenced my bleeding cycle. This term actually dates back thousands of years. The Greek roots *peri* and *hodos* are the source for *period* and signify both time and way. The Latin *periodos* means "cycle," specifically a cycle that repeats. I wish that I would have known the simple elegance of that reference in my teens, but I did not.

In the last thirty or so years, I've developed the habit of tracing words that I want to be in deeper relationship with, exploring them back to their root and core. I have come to both value and adore etymology as an adult. Understanding this sensible origin of the term *period* gives me a greater respect for the labeling of my cycle. As a young woman, I had not begun the habit of sitting with words yet, and *period* as a term was not explained in health class or by my community, so it seemed a bit arbitrary to me. Rather, it was the term *menstruation* that was used in education. Like so many of our Western scientific terms, *menstruation* is sourced from Latin—*menstruus*—and simply means "monthly." All of which is to bring you along with me to the term that I have used since my early twenties to refer to my monthly bleed, *moon time*. I first heard the term *moon time* used in the Piscataway community in southern Maryland. The Piscataway are indigenous to North America and were one of several tribes that lived on the Chesapeake Bay and surrounding regions of what are now named Maryland, Delaware, and Virginia. Being in relationship with the Piscataway Indian Nation and invited to sweat lodges and the Sun Dance ceremony in Tayac Territory set my life in a very specific direction. It was here that I began to love my body and the ways of my body and here that prayer felt alive in my body. It was also in this community that I was surrounded by friends who made me feel genuinely seen, because they loved the Earth as deeply and reverently as I did. It is a powerful thing, to be seen and accepted for who you are; it is a potent and compelling invitation to trust and prioritize the relationship with your own soul.

The women in the community that surrounded the Piscataway Indian Nation (both Native and non-Native) were thoroughly engaged in fairly conventional lifestyles but also steeped in teachings handed down through maternal lines. Here, for the first time, my moon time was viewed as a reminder of my power, as a sacred and beautiful rhythm to embrace. In this community, I learned to step away from the larger community when bleeding—not because I was dirty, impure, or weak but because I was full of power. This community of women knew to draw inward and nourish themselves at this time; in doing so, they nourished their power. During a woman's moon time, she will not sweat in sweat lodges with men nor will she come onto the grounds of a Sun Dance ceremony, because her prayer at this time is so mighty and so compelling that it will drown out every other prayer. Instead, women use this as a time to deepen and strengthen relationships to other women as well as to more deeply listen to the counsel of the moon.

For these reasons, *moon time* is the term that resonates for me and many women. I respectfully acknowledge that I live, learn, and love on the lands of the Eastern Band of Cherokee as well as the lands of the Yuchi people. To use the term *moon time* for my monthly blood feels, in some microcosmic way, like a means to express respect for and bow to the women whose land I live on. I would encourage you to find a way to think of and refer to your monthly bleed that resonates for you and reminds you of the power and potential of your monthly cycle. Remember that we believe every single thing that we tell ourselves, and we talk to ourselves in an almost steady stream: to rename this cycle in a way that feels reverent and respectful to us is one of many things we can do as women to reclaim our power.

The term *moon time* also acknowledges the connection of our bodies' cycles of menstrual waxing and waning with that of the moon's cycle of waxing and waning. Does our cycle link to the moon? Research studies correlate a relationship as often as they dispute it. What I have been taught, as well as what I have witnessed in my own life, is that there is indeed a correlation. In modern times of electric light and glowing screens and other influences that leave us out of sync with nature, to be linked to the moon through your cycle is increasingly rare. When I first began to bleed, I tended to ovulate around the full moon and bleed around the new moon. After high school, I delayed college and went traveling for a bit; but when I went to college, I lost my original cycle. My guess is that it had a lot to do with staying up late and staying in various homes that did not afford natural darkness—along with the light of my own indoor living space, including television and computer screens, darkness was kept at bay by street and city lights outside of the places where I lived.

My monthly cycle did, however, sync up with the cycles of women whom I lived with. Have you ever noticed this in your own life? Often, when women live together, their cycles will synchronize. Our maternal ancestors noticed this as well, and numerous rituals around the world are a result of women bleeding in community. Once I left college and settled down in the Appalachian Mountains, far away from any city, let alone visible neighbors, my cycle returned again to ovulating around the full moon and bleeding around the new moon. As I left the childbirth years and began the journey to my wise woman years, my cycle shifted yet again—to ovulating on the new moon and bleeding at the full moon.

Studies have corroborated this apparent deep connection to the moon—for instance, finding that peak rates of conception occur at the time of the full moon and conception rates fall at the new moon. We are our ancestors; they are our very DNA. Long before the advent of the industrial age, in simpler times and all over the world, communities would gather around or on the full moon. The light of the moon made travel of multiple days much easier. It makes sense that our biology would tend toward fertility increasing at a time when there would be more opportunity to partner. This same logic applies to bleeding at the new moon, when there was no light and the nights were long and dark. It would be more desirable to stay in—easier to hunker down and allow our bodies to release and bleed.

The moon rules the ocean tides; it's no surprise that it likewise has a powerful effect on reproductive cycles and fertility. But the moon also affects our moods, and it even seems to visit our unconscious mind, impacting our sleep and our dreams. Numerous scientific studies note a correlation between sleeping and dreaming cycles and moon phases, with the full moon by far having the greatest impact. It would be easy to attribute this to the increased light, but studies have compensated for that by having participants sleep in completely darkened rooms as well as by not revealing the purpose of the study while it was underway. The outcomes suggest that we are deeply attuned to the moon, whether we see her or have an awareness of her or not.

In various women's circles that I have been in over the years, time and time again, someone has brought up the notion of a red moon cycle and a white moon cycle. The white moon cycle is when you ovulate at the full moon and bleed at the new moon. This cycle is thought to be more fertile. The red moon cycle is the reverse—where ovulation happens around the new moon and bleeding at the full moon. This cycle also holds fertility—but that fertility seems to involve creativity and projects and nourishing others. Again, with consideration, this duality of cycles makes sense: not all women choose to birth children, but they may instead birth other things—from businesses to art to gardens to teaching projects to healing projects and far too many other wondrous things to name! As well, in ancient cultures where bleeding women might have withdrawn from daily life and concerns, it would have been other women, those not bleeding, who would have been in a position to keep the link between the two worlds—from bringing sustenance to a moon lodge to showing up in the community while many of the women were in renewal.

As you track your own moon time, you may notice a correlation with the phases of the moon or you may not. All of our cycles are different. Some of us bleed for three days, some for five. The number of days in your cycle matters less than whether it is regular: consistent, predictable, and known to you. Stress, tension, shock, and trauma can all knock our moon time out of schedule, but if our underlying condition is one of health, our pattern will return. Should you find that you are not in any discernable relationship to the moon phases and you wish to be, you can see what happens when you spend consistent time outside in nature. It can also be enormously beneficial to reduce your hours of artificial light in the evenings. Sleeping in true dark with no nightlights or screen lights can enhance whole body wellness and also our circadian rhythms. A consistent schedule of waking and sleeping can also benefit your overall health and rhythm and harmony with the larger cycles of moon, Earth, and sun.

THE MOON MOVES THROUGH YOUR BODY: THE MOON CENTER CYCLE

The second moon cycle that happens within us has to do with the way the moon moves through our bodies. This "moon center cycle" belongs to all who identify as woman; it is formed while we are still in utero and it stays with us for our entire lives. Our moon center cycle is our own (unique to us) coding of the journey of the moon during our formation.

As the moon traverses the constellations on her elliptical orbit around the Earth, she is also spinning on her axis. Notably, both the orbit around Earth and the axis rotation take 27.3 days. As the moon is spinning and orbiting Earth, Earth is also rotating on its axis and revolving around the sun. The sun rotates as well, but because it is basically a big exploding ball of gas (the nature of stars), the rotation is quite different. The sun rotates faster in the center (that is, at its equator), taking about 27 days, and slower at the poles, taking about 31 days. That in itself is somewhat fantastical.

Circles upon circles—moons (satellites) orbiting planets, planets orbiting the sun, and the sun slowly and steadily revolving around the center of the Milky Way galaxy (thought to take around 250 million years)—along with magnetic fields, solar flares, tidal bulges, gravitational pull, and the travels of light are all part of this grand architecture that creates us. And yet, more than any other feature, the moon exerts the most profound influence on us. Our moon center cycle is one of the many gifts the moon bestows upon us.

This moon center cycle is analogous to a map, in two ways. First, it is the ethereal footprint of the moon's journey through the sky while we were in utero. Second, once we discern our moon center cycle, we unlock a map to ourselves, finding a pattern to our own tides of emotion and longing and behavior.

I first learned about the moon center cycle teachings when I began to practice kundalini yoga. I was much younger and had not been doing yoga for long. I was seeking to replicate an experience I had practicing with a teacher in California when I stumbled into a kundalini ashram in Washington, D.C. Both the ashram and kundalini yoga were different from anything I had ever encountered. The practice felt like coming home, yet the home was nowhere I had ever been before, at least in this lifetime. Again, I had the sensation of prayer alive in my body. Since that first class in 1990, yoga has profoundly shaped my days, months, life, relationships, and beliefs.

Kundalini yoga is deeply tantric in philosophy and execution. Kundalini practitioners are not celibate but rather are considered householders—living in the world, earning a living, creating family—and kundalini practices are not only for the individual. Many practices from this tradition are also for relationship, for family, for ancestors, for community.

Kundalini is an ancient practice that continues to offer relevant guidance in today's world. The exact origin of the moon center cycle teachings has been obscured by time, or secrecy, or both. Given the reverence that these teachings accord to the moon and to the cycles of nature and the feminine, it is plausible that they are tantric in origin—yet they might also come from the Bronze Age Indus-Sarasvati Civilization more generally. This was the largest civilization of antiquity, named for the Indus and Sarasvati river valleys of Bharatvarsha (present-day India and Pakistan) and its development began over twelve thousand years ago. Worship of nature, of the moon and sun, and of Shakti (the feminine embodiment and source of all creation) is apparent from excavated artifacts. It was here too, possibly some five thousand years ago, that the practice of yoga began.

The teachings of the moon center cycles begin with knowing that all of us have one moon center in our chin, and this where we receive the energy of the moon. For those of us who identify as being predominately solar, shaped more by the sun than the moon (some would say masculine), there is only this one moon center. For those of us who identify as more lunar, there are an additional eleven centers where the moon energy entwines with us and shapes our bodies, our emotion, our perspective. And through these twelve centers, the moon moves through our bodies.

While I consider kundalini yoga to be the *maha* (great) practice of my heart, I also identify as a "yoga universalist"—someone who loves all the traditions and styles. My interpretation of the way the moon travels through the centers of a woman's body differs slightly from the standard presentation in the kundalini community. The traditional kundalini interpretation acknowledges the chin center but only has the moon moving through the eleven centers of the body. My presentation has the moon spending time in the chin as well, and it aligns much more organically with the journey of the moon through the sky as well as with Vedic astrology.

As previously mentioned, the moon's elliptical orbit around Earth takes 27.3 days—yet as you'll notice when we dive into the third cycle for consideration, moon phases, it takes the moon 29.5 days to complete her phases. As a result of Earth's revolution around the sun, the moon has to rotate just a little bit more to get back in the same position. Often, you'll hear the moon's cycle averaged between the two (27.3 and 29.5) and stated as 28 days between lunations—that is, from new moon to new moon. As the moon journeys the sky, we feel her energy in a unique pattern in each of our twelve moon centers. Just as the moon energy is moving through one constellation for about 2.3 days, she also spends 2.3 days in one of the twelve moon centers of our bodies. The movement of the moon in our bodies is incredibly subtle and takes time to discern. Also, each woman's moon center pattern (the way the moon progresses through the moon centers) is different. Allowing yourself the time to detect and distinguish the pattern with which the moon moves through your body is a powerful and incredibly deep way to be in relationship with yourself.

Women might wear an air of mystery to others, but we should never be a mystery to ourselves. Determining your unique pattern of moon center movement will unlock the rhythm to your moods and your behavior as well as give you an understanding of your flow of energy, of your tendencies toward both need and want during a lunation. Knowing yourself so intimately is also a way to unlock incredible potential in your life.

When the moon is in one of the twelve moon centers in your body, it shows up in a certain way and influences you in specific ways. Your most important tools in discerning your unique pattern of moon center movement are deep inner listening, patience, and intuition. It generally takes between three and four months to begin to find your pattern.

As you learn to identify the moon center of your body where the moon is dwelling, you will also see certain characteristics that appear in your way of interacting with the world. The list of the body's twelve moon centers, below, also notes the ways in which we could feel and be driven while the moon is in that center. This list is meant to be broad-ranging and allow for a spectrum of potentiality. In discerning your pattern, you might find that one suggestion is very helpful and others are not. Trust yourself. This pattern has been with you as long as you have been you, and you are simply drawing back the veil on what that pattern is.

PENDULUMS

Some women have found success using pendulums to both find and confirm their pattern. Pendulums are utilized for questions that can be answered yes or no. Any object hanging from a chain or a string can be used, but pendulums are often very purposefully made, with the dangling object holding meaning for the owner. The object used could be something like a crystal, a coin, or a stone, or it could be made from wood or glass or metal. You can also purchase rather than make a pendulum. Regardless of the source, seek to use a pendulum that speaks to you in some way—be it aesthetic or compelling for some other reason—because when you pose a question to a pendulum, you are really asking for the answer from your inner knowing or higher self. The pendulum is a tool for connecting with the energy of you.

Before working with your pendulum, create a ritual of cleansing it. It can be nice to wash it in cool water and allow it to soak up the light of the full moon. You could also burn mugwort or rosemary and allow the smoke to cleanse the pendulum. White sage has a long history of being used for purification but some medicinal plant conservationists warn that its harvest for such purposes is unsustainable. Furthermore, it is considered sacred by many Indigenous people—to be used for medicinal and ceremonial use only. Put simply, to burn white sage outside of those ceremonies is unethical and amounts to cultural appropriation.

Once your pendulum is clean, find a quiet space and time and allow your mind to become more meditative. Take the end of the pendulum chain (or string) with your dominant hand and allow it to dangle freely. Ask the pendulum to show you "yes" and note which way the pendulum moves. Ask to see "no" and again note the movement. If this is your first time using a pendulum, you could ask some questions that are yes or no that you already know the answers to, as a confirmation that you understand the movements. Then, simply meditate on the moon and where she might be in your body. When you have an idea of a specific center, ask the pendulum if the moon is there. Ideally, you will have done some charting or journaling along these lines already (see page 000) and have an idea of where the moon is moving. You should also plan to only ask one question per sitting. Remember that the moon moves every 2.3 days, so the amount of time that the moon is in a center is defined.

1. CHIN. Feelings of stability, affection, care. A pull toward the new and original as well as the unconventional. Curiosity around new technology, innovation. A good time to explore new horizons, to learn new things, to give rein to personal freedom and expression. Sensations of feeling positively anchored.

2. LIPS. A strong desire to communicate, both in expression and analyzing. Emotions are balanced and calm, yet not fixed. The mind is clear and fast; this speed of thought can pour into talking, so remember to listen as well. Motivated. A good time to connect intellectually. Reception to insights and epiphanies and a desire to share them as well.

3. CHEEKS. Emotional state is heightened with impulsive energy. Can feel extreme. Self-focused and quick actions and reactions. Slightly aggressive swirls and impulses. Desire to assert self, especially through the lens of your own sensitivities. Restlessness. Physical exercise can be a great outlet at this time. The most compelling compass is internal, yet awareness of the bigger picture is always appropriate.

4. EARLOBES. Concentrated and controlled. Ease in balance between home and work. Prudent, conservative. Impersonal thinking. Self-disciplined. Good self-control. Ambitious. This is a time to avoid rigidity, and this energy can be utilized for planning out those hard and continuous things in life. Sustained energy, especially when consciously directed.

5. EYEBROWS. Things feel shrouded in mystery and obscurity. Can feel dreamy as well as have an inclination toward fantasy. Might feel overly sensitive and experience a difficulty in concentrating. Emotions beckon your attention more strongly than logic or thinking. This can be a good time to seek solitude and time with art or music. Feeling all the feels. Riding the waves is more useful than interpreting them at this time.

6. ARCLINE (hairline). Emotions feel on an even keel. Can feel borderline aggressive in pursuit of perfection. Critical of self and others. Affinity with skill, precision, attention to detail. Desire for organization. This can be a good time to clean and cleanse. Very much in the present moment. An excellent time to apply yourself to any projects that benefit from attention to detail.

7. BACK OF NECK. Call to beauty, to intimacy, to the romantic. Heightened sense of material assets, money issues. Enhanced endurance. The sensual aspects of life are noticed and appreciated. Home and family beckon. A desire to eat more

could show up. This is a good time to make aesthetic changes to the self or the environment. Appreciating art, talent, and skill is easeful now.

8. BREASTS. This is a watery center for the moon and a sense of homecoming might be present. There is a sense of belonging, of care, of protection. We can feel tender, compassionate, very loving. We can desire understanding as well as security. A desire to nourish. Anything that needs nurturing benefits from your attention now.

9. NAVEL. A desire to express oneself. Can feel called to create, build, highlight as well as a desire to call attention to oneself, possibly prideful. A yearning to have our qualities recognized. Radiance and personal will feel strong and centered. A sense of self-sufficiency. Watch for vanity. This is a good time to relax and let go. There is an enhanced ability to put things into perspective, especially the judgments of others.

10. VAGINA. Depth. Everything feels deep. Currents come to the surface, subconscious as well as intuition. Ability to understand the often unexplainable, the mysterious. Intense emotions and feelings. A desire to share and connect. Passionate and amplified. This juncture offers us the clearest opportunity for self-revelation.

11. CLITORIS. Strong positive feelings and sense of optimism, vitality. Desire to move and travel. Fresh information often comes to light; a good opportunity to listen for what is important. Spontaneous, riding the wave. Good time to use this energy to release negativity. Another good time in the cycle to cleanse, less physically and more energetically.

12. INNER THIGHS. A desire to both confirm and affirm. Good balance between personal needs and the needs of those closest to you. Can feel a little impulsive but the desire for balance and harmony is what is strongest. A desire for justice, impartiality. Mutuality and intimacy. Harmony within self, within skin. Can feel difficult to make decisions due to the ability to see both (or all) sides.

To begin to track the movement of the moon in your body, make notes on what you are feeling each day—habitually in the morning and evening if you can, but also at any point during the day if you feel or recognize something strongly within you. You could use the reproducible chart on page 37 for this or simply a notebook. These notes could be just a word or two, maybe more, but keep it short. You are looking to recognize patterns rather than create a diary of your life.

Although your moon center cycle is created while you are still in the womb of your mother, trauma or shock can shift your cycle. If you find that you are missing a center or two—you don't feel quite confident in what you are feeling or its energy—consider the possibility that some event, as a child or an adult, changed the way the moon feels in that center. Again, the most important thing in this learning of your cycle is trust in yourself, in your intuition and your own inner wisdom. Sometimes your moon center cycle will return eventually to the original, unique pattern you were born with after a shock, but sometimes not. Even if you are not quite sure of your pattern yet, you can balance your moon centers by using a variation of the **Kirtan Kriya** meditation in chapter 5 (pages 88–89).

Your moon center cycle stays with you for your entire life. To understand, for example, when you might feel most ambitious or most sensitive, or when you might desire an intellectual connection, is a powerful insight in to your own self. Knowing your patterns can help you to utilize your greatest strength in this lifetime. That strength is the unique gift that you and you alone are.

MOON PHASES

The truest lunar cycle would include the dark moon, a place in the cycle just before the new moon shows its sliver of light, when it is void of light and yet deeply rich with the potential for the illumination of integrated wisdom. Our ancestors knew the dark moon, understanding in their bones that it was a pause, a completion. It represents both integration and emptying, in the same way that we take the pose of the corpse at the end of our practice, allowing the practice to integrate through our many layers of being, while also emptying ourselves of effort, thought, and striving.

The dark moon is when zero percent of the moon's surface is illuminated (identifying the surface percentage illuminated, rather than naming the phase, is a more precise way to consider the way the moon looks at different points in the cycle), and it lasts just less than twenty-four hours—the percentage of light that the moon reflects is always increasing or decreasing, depending upon where in the cycle we are. You will easily find the exact time of the dark moon in astronomical charts, although the term they use will be *new moon*. I'm not quite sure how or when the "dark" moon became the "new" moon: plentiful references to the dark moon appear in the nineteenth-century sources, and modern dictionary definitions of the new moon still define that stage as it was understood by our ancestors—as the time when the moon has a faint visible crescent of light.

As the natural world teaches, the end feeds into the beginning and the beginning takes us all the way around to the end, over and over. And we see the same with the moon. From the sliver of illumination that announces the new moon, we roll into the waxing crescent moon, a time where the sliver of light is increasing, growing to the first quarter moon, where half of the moon is illuminated. Viewed from the Northern Hemisphere, the right side of the moon looks bright and the left side dark. That is reversed in the Southern Hemisphere. Our moon continues to grow, and about two weeks from the dark moon, we arrive at the waxing gibbous moon, almost full. Next is the full moon, the peak of illumination, when the Earth is between the sun and the moon. From this apex of light, the light of the moon begins to diminish, and this is the waning gibbous moon, more than halfway lit but no longer full. The next phase is the last quarter moon, where half of the moon is in darkness and half is in light. And then, the moon reaches the phase of waning crescent, the light slowly waning until there is just a sliver of a crescent of light left. This phase takes us to the end of the lunation, the dark moon.

Astronomers consider the four primary phases to be new moon, first quarter moon, full moon, and last quarter moon, as these are exact and precise moments in the lunar cycle. The waxing crescent, waxing gibbous, waning gibbous, and waning crescent phases are considered secondary or intermediary phases, as these are spans of time rather than clearly defined moments.

DOES OUR MOON HAVE EIGHT PHASES OR NINE?

We might question whether our moon has eight phases or nine, and the question itself points to a lovely shroud of flux, flow, and mystery—much like the embodiment of being woman. An astronomer will tell you the phases are eight, and yet, for me, it's important to include the dark moon in both ritual and recognition. As it is modern-day astronomy that substituted "new moon" for "dark moon" while picking up the thread of our ancestors' wisdom and instituting it on calendars and scientifically, I think that you get to decide for yourself. Think about what feels most resonant to you in your relationship to the moon. Best of all, this can even be in flux and flow—it may be that some months you feel the dark moon keenly, and other months, it is all about the new moon. Keeping a journal of thoughts, emotions, desires, and hopes through the month, as well as naming our needs, is one more way not only to come into a deeper relationship with ourselves but also to deepen our relationship to the moon. Below is a recap of the moon's phases, in order, from beginning to end, with descriptions of the associated energy.

NEW MOON. A primary phase and precise moment in time. (See "Dark moon," below.) The energy of the new moon invites *us* to begin again, as well. This "begin again," or sowing of seeds, is most potent about twenty-four hours out from the astronomical new moon.

WAXING CRESCENT. A secondary phase, the span of time bridging the new moon and the first quarter, where the illumination of the moon is faint at the start but increasing. If we continue our gardening analogy, this is the sprouting period, a time of intention.

FIRST QUARTER. Primary phase, the precise moment when the moon is a quarter of the way through the cycle (one-fourth of the way through the circular orbit around Earth) and halfway illuminated. This is a time of action—think of how a sprouting plant might meet obstacles and you've got it! Resistances, whether internal or external, give us an opportunity to apply ourselves in the right direction.

WAXING GIBBOUS. Secondary phase, with the light headed to full illumination. Here is where we can course correct, refine, and edit our action energy.

FULL MOON. A primary phase, precisely noted in time no matter where on Earth you are. This is the peak of light and also energy. Bathed in full illumination, we have our clearest perception and we can choose to harvest or release.

WANING GIBBOUS. A secondary phase, with the light now diminishing. We can choose the energy of gratitude and appreciation for this time and for our harvest (even release is a reaping of sorts).

LAST QUARTER. Primary phase again, in which the light has dwindled from full to half and the moon is three-quarters of the way through her journey. What do we need to release? What do we let go of to lighten the load? Here is the gift of choosing what to compost.

WANING CRESCENT. The home stretch, and a secondary phase again. This is the final time of jettisoning, as we surrender to what we know comes next, beginning the move to rest.

DARK MOON. The time of the cycle embraced by our ancestors as void. The gift of the dark moon is liminal; it is the bottom of the exhale as we move into rest and release. In this state, integration is possible. As very few calendars or modern cultures recognize the way the moon occupies this place, consider giving yourself a day of rest and release on the day marked as the new moon, holding this day as sacred pause. Twenty-four hours after your deep and sacred rest (basically the next day), allow yourself to begin to percolate the new—the energy of initiation as you step toward the new moon and the luminous journey begins anew.

THE MOON IS SOVEREIGN, WITHIN AND WITHOUT, A REMINDER OF CONNECTION AND POWER

The moon invites our relationship to her in powerful ways, from the witnessing of her phases and passage to the way she shows up in our bodies. She connects us in deep and powerful ways to earth, to nature, and to cosmic forces. We do not need to search for our connection to nature; rather we are reminded every few days, every month, of our sacred and holy bond. When we feel outside of connection, we can always look up to the sky and find her, speak with her.

Tantra teaches that the universe has come forward from the womb of Kali, the goddess of creation, of time, of power and destruction. Tantra also holds that the moon time and blood are *pushpa*—"the flower." Flowers are the sexual organs of plants, announcing fertility and enticing creation. The very magic of creation actually resides in our moon blood. Tantric traditions and Hindu traditions alike teach that as Kali created the universe, woman creates life.

Our moon times and moon center cycles are no curse; they are power and connection. While they may contribute to an air of mystery attached to those who identify as women, deeply understanding our lunar nature dissolves any inscrutability we might have in relationship to ourselves, to our own soul. And more broadly, to look to the sky and know the moon is to connect not only with that lunar body but also with our ancestors; in some small and sweet way, we connect to everyone who has ever looked at the moon with love and awe and a desire to know her.

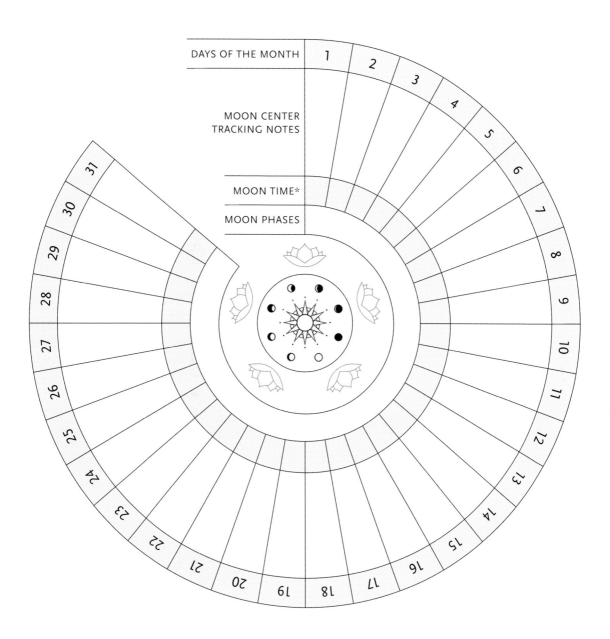

DAYS OF THE MONTH

MOON CENTER
TRACKING NOTES

MOON TIME*

MOON PHASES

1 2 3 4 5 6 7 8 9 10 11 12 13 14 15 16 17 18 19 20 21 22 23 24 25 26 27 28 29 30 31

*Bleeding Cycles

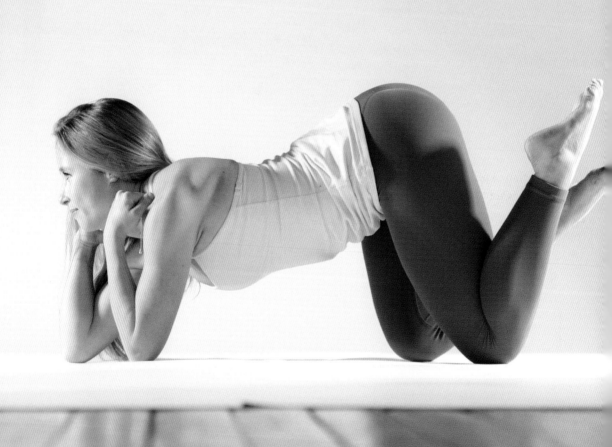

4

Practices for Moon Times

T O A CERTAIN EXTENT, the entire month is a moon time for us in one way or another. While the moon takes 27.3 days to travel the Earth orbit, her cycle is 29.5 days, from beginning to end. Our moon spends those extra days making up the difference between her orbit around the Earth and the Earth's orbit around the sun. Often, the cycle is averaged, referred to as 28 days.

Chapter 3 outlined the four primary phases of the moon's monthly cycle as well as her four secondary phases. In this chapter, we consider the possible correlation between the moon's four general stages (new, waxing, full, and waning) and the four phases of menstruation.

In bodies that bleed, the first day that we bleed is considered day 1 of our ovarian and uterine cycles. This bleeding phase of the uterine cycle is known as menstruation, a phase where we are shedding the thickened lining of the uterus. Our moon blood is a fluid of blood, cells from the lining of the uterus, and mucus. Every woman is a little different in the amount of time that she bleeds, usually between three and seven days. The second, overlapping phase of moon time, the follicular phase, also begins on the first day of bleeding but it continues longer—until we ovulate. During the follicular phase, the pituitary gland is releasing follicle-stimulating hormone, which stimulates the ovaries to produce anywhere between five and twenty follicles. Each ovarian follicle contains an immature egg, and the growth of these follicles signals the start of the menstrual cycle and stimulates the lining of the uterus to thicken. This thickening is the way the body prepares for possible pregnancy. Usually only one follicle ripens into a mature egg and the rest of the follicles die and are reabsorbed. This happens around day 10 or so of the ovarian cycle. The remaining follicle begins to produce large amounts of estrogen and, on approximately day 14, a hormone surge triggers the next phase.

With the end of the follicular phase comes ovulation, the next or third phase, when a mature egg is released from the surface of the ovary, about midway through the cycle. Here, the egg is channeled into the fallopian tube and toward the uterus. The egg only has a life span of about twenty-four hours; unless egg and sperm meet during this process, the egg will die. After ovulation, we enter a fourth phase, the luteal phase. The follicle that released the egg transforms into what is known as the *corpus luteum*. (*Corpus*, of course, means "body," and *luteum* refers to the composition of this body—lutein cells. Luteum and lutein are both derived from the Latin *luteus*, which means saffron yellow! The corpus luteum tissue is temporary and considered to be an endocrine structure.)

In the body's luteal phase, the hormones testosterone, progesterone, and estrogen are at peak levels, rebuilding the uterine lining. If egg and sperm meet and the egg is fertilized and implants in the uterine lining, the hormones necessary for continued growth are produced and this is the start of pregnancy. If the egg is not fertilized, then the corpus luteum shrivels around the twenty-second day of the cycle. This causes a drop in progesterone. and again, we return to the phase of releasing blood.

It's a bit of magic and connection to consider the phases of menstruation and the moon phases as kin. Some wisdom traditions align these phases—drawing a correlation between the new moon and menstruation. Both of these phases, whether aligned or not, have elements of rest and initiation. The follicular phase and the waxing moon are aligned in sharing the elements of stimulation, building, and increasing. During the bleeding years, we might also feel this expansion in the ways we engage in our social life as well as our working life. Ovulation and the full moon are linked as the peak of the cycle and energy. While many of us do ovulate at the full moon, many of us do not. See if you can create room in your life to be aware of the peak energy of ovulation within, as it happens, regardless of which phase the moon is in. The luteal phase and the waning of the moon are energetically associated, as our bodies are in preparation for the possible creation of life and the moon is drawing down and entering darkness in preparation for her own new life. This is a lovely time of our cycle as well as the moon's cycle to engage in soothing practices.

You might find that the phases of your moon time cycle align with the phases of the moon, but then again you might not! This is an area chock-full of valid research that both supports and disputes an alignment. Some wisdom traditions, especially the more orthodox lineages of Ayurveda, advocate that we work to sync ourselves to the moon and her phases as a way of restoring health. I tend to part ways from this stance and believe that what we need for health is much more nuanced and complex than simply syncing our menstruation. Life itself has become ever more complex for us, and we negotiate terrain that our ancestors would not have even been able to imagine. Again, a menstrual cycle that is regular and manifests with a sameness and familiarity to you each month, regardless of moon phase, is a much truer indication of health, in my humble opinion.

Perhaps in wilder times, long ago, all bodies with monthly bleeds were aligned in sync with the moon, and perhaps not. Regardless, it has always been both resonant and helpful to me to be aware of both the astronomical moon phase and my own moon time phase. This awareness has enabled me to provide myself both with deeper self-care and with deeper self-compassion as I have come to understand that my energy as well as my resilience is impacted by the phases of both cycles.

The four practices included at the end of this chapter are shared in the hope that you will find ways to care for yourself as you traverse the month. These practices can be done in accordance with moon phases, in harmony with your own menstrual phases, or simply because the practice and energy are calling to you.

The **Gentle Restorative Practice** is appropriate for bleeding days. On our bleeding days, inversions—such as handstands, headstands, Plow Pose, Shoulderstand, and the like—are discouraged as are any practices that are super-strenuous or draw upon core strength unduly. It is also advised to refrain from engaging mula bandha, the root lock. The reason for these cautions is based on the flow of prana in our bodies and aligning our practice to take advantage of the inherent nature of prana and flow. Inversions place our bodies in direct conflict with *apana*, one of the five primary life forces, or pranic winds referenced in the Tips, Tools, and Illuminations section. These pranic winds are more accurately known as *vayus*. The term *vayu* translates to "wind" or "gale" and refers to the homes that the maha prana take up in our bodies. There are five primary vayus in the body, and prana takes on specific attributes, characteristics, and functions based on the vayu. The five primary vayus are udana, prana, samana, apana, and vyana. Of these five primary pranas, two are dominant: *prana prana*, located at the heart—an upward and filling, intaking prana—and *apana prana*, which lives in the pelvic bowl, down to the feet—a downward energy, emptying and carrying away. Apana is the prana that supports the downward flow and release of menstrual blood and is the reason for the teachings that ask us to refrain from inversions while bleeding. The inherent function of apana is also the reason that we refrain from engaging mula bandha when we are bleeding; to engage this lock is to pull up and hold that which we wish to release at that time. If you have left your bleeding years or live in a body that has never had a blood cycle, the **Gentle Restorative Practice** can be sweet on low-energy days or around the time of the new moon, when we often feel tired.

MORE ON MOON TIME PRACTICE

The teachings of not practicing inversions, or mula bandha, during bleeding days are ancient and have been handed down through generations as a way of respecting the flow of prana in our bodies. The Ayurvedic perspective would not only advise against inversions but also against practicing at all on bleeding days. Regarding the actual moon phases, some classic yogic traditions encourage observing the "moon days"—usually meaning the full moon and the new moon, but in some cases also the dark moon day and the eleventh day of the moon—by abstaining from the physical practice of yoga. The Ashtanga tradition is one school of yoga that still follows this counsel. Ashtanga is a physically demanding form of practice. This tradition asks us to practice all of the eight limbs of the beginner path on our mat, simultaneously, as we move through the asanas. Other traditions do not advocate for abstention from practice on full or new moon days but instead recognize the power and influence of the moon by invoking the moon in some way during practice—whether in meditation, posture, pranayama, or simple devotion.

Ultimately, what is most important is listening to your body and practicing in a way that feels true for you. Choosing to align your practice to your own phase or to the moon phase, as well as choosing whether to practice or not on moon days, is truly up to your discretion and an opportunity to embrace your inner wisdom and allow your sovereign self to shine.

Kriya to Support Apana and Elimination is the next practice offered and is brilliant for supporting our apana prana force in the body as well as elimination in general. Our digestive system needs healthy elimination to function, and this kriya supports the physical aspects of elimination as well as the more esoteric aspects of release: letting go of toxic emotions or stress. With the exception of the heaviest days of bleeding, this kriya can be practiced any time you wish to work with the energy of elimination.

Body Beautiful is a lovely sweet and short practice that I go to again and again, both for its simplicity as well as its lack of contraindications. A pleasant container for full moon energy can be created when this practice is combined with Moon Salutations.

The **Sequence to Relieve PMS—or to Slow Down and Experience Gratitude** is the final practice in this chapter. Not all women experience premenstrual syndrome, and PMS can be somewhat medically vague, with upward of a hundred different symptoms possible, all of which are unpleasant (headaches, bloating, cramping, and so on). Generally, experiencing three to five of the symptoms regularly, prior to menstruating, is considered PMS. PMS is thought to be caused by a combination of imbalanced hormones and a sluggish liver. This sequence has an element of challenge to it and is a good way to shift into a place that is unhurried and to allow ourselves the time and space to dwell on our gratitudes, all that we appreciate, whether we suffer from PMS or not.

GENTLE RESTORATIVE PRACTICE

This flow can be embellished and reordered in any sequence that you wish and is especially well received by the body in times when rest and restoration are sought.

Consider beginning with some conscious breath work, depending upon the qualities of energy you seek. A segmented breath, breaking the inhale into four equal sections, or "sniffs," and exhaling in one long continuous breath, offers energy and boosts mood. A segmented breath of four equal parts to the inhale and eight equal parts to the exhale offers a sense of calm and seemingly dissolves energy blocks, helping us to let go.

More than any other practice in this book, the experience in the **Gentle Restorative Practice** can be greatly enhanced by the use of props—yoga bolsters, blocks, blankets, maybe some pillows.

1. Sit on your heels and shift your knees to have them a bit wider than your hips. From here, rest your torso forward. Relax your head on the earth and allow your arms to relax back alongside your legs, palms facing up. A bolster or some blankets in front of you, just between your knees, can create more access and more comfort. If using a bolster, you may find it more comfortable to relax your arms forward from the shoulders, with your forearms and palms resting on the earth. Turn your head to one side and allow a long, deep breath. Close your eyes, or soften your gaze to no focus. Spend about 5 minutes in this pose, turning your head in the other direction halfway through. When finished, take your time coming back up out of the pose and transition slowly.

2. Lie down and lengthen your back along the floor. Bend your knees, placing your feet hip-width apart. Your head is relaxed on the floor, as are your shoulders and arms. Lift your hips and slide a yoga block or substitute (firm pillow, folded blankets, even a stack of books) under your hips, at the tailbone, then release down. Once your hips are supported, allow your palms to turn upward and tuck your chin the tiniest bit to lengthen the back of your neck. Allow your eyes to close or soften. Find your breath and relax here for about 5 minutes. When finished, lift your hips, slide the prop out from under, and slowly come upright.

3. Once upright, sit with your legs spread comfortably wide. Bring a bolster (or substitute) toward your torso, in between your legs. Lean forward from the hips, initially keeping your back straight, and then relax your head down onto the support, resting your forehead there. (If there is access and comfort for this shape without props, feel free to skip them. In that case, your forehead rests on floor.) Begin to release and relax through your neck, shoulders, and chest. Gradually relax your entire body. Find a deep, slow breath. Relax here for approximately 5 minutes. Gently ease yourself up from the posture.

▷

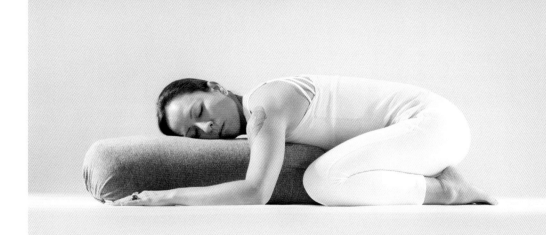

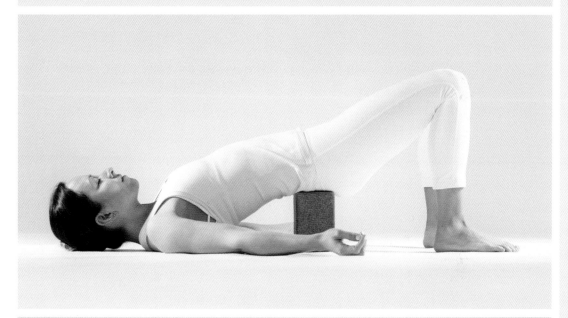

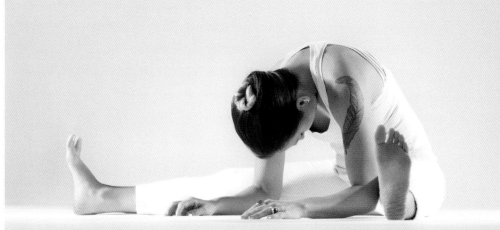

4. Move to a wall, then sitting with one side to the wall, gradually ease down onto your back and turn to bring your legs up to rest on the wall. Your legs should be relaxed and supported, rather than perfectly straight. Your arms relax along the side of your body, palms turned skyward. Unwind here, with slow deep breathing (see page 5) for 5 minutes. This posture is restorative for the adrenals and excellent for times when you feel maxed out. If it isn't possible to place your legs up a wall, you can rest them up and over a chair, bolsters, or a mound of pillows for the same effect.

5. Star-shaped Shavasana, or Corpse Pose, is the final posture and place of integration. Prepare two blankets, rolling each into a tube shape. Relax back and allow your legs to open in a V shape. Place one of the blankets horizontally so that it is under the backs of both knees. Place the other blanket just under the base of your cranium, at the back of your neck. Your arms finish the shape of the star, relaxed gently out (lower than shoulder level) to the sides. Feel the support of the earth, feel the blankets, and knowing you are held, relax your entire body. Take 7–10 minutes here, maybe even a little nap! When finished, while still on your back, stretch a bit, in all directions.

6. If you like, you could also finish with a bit of breath work, using one of the breaths outlined above, or you could choose to end with a meditation.

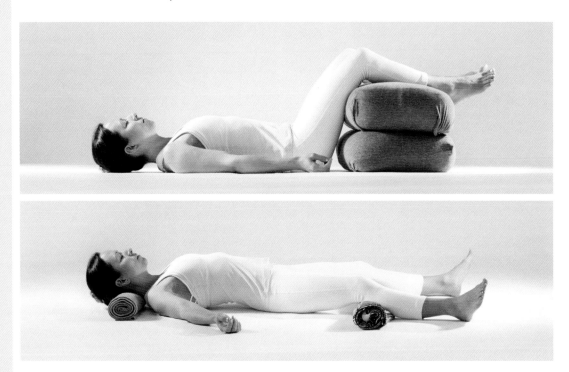

KRIYA TO SUPPORT APANA AND ELIMINATION

This kriya supports the digestive system and the overall eliminative ability of our physical body. Enhanced eliminative energy also supports our ability to release emotional and energetic burdens. Avoid this practice on your heaviest bleeding days.

1. We begin with Vatskar Kriya (a kriya within a kriya!). Vatskar Kriya alone (without continuing for the rest of this sequence here) is considered a complete practice for the digestion. It is important to do this on an empty stomach. Sit in Sukhasana resting your hands on your knees. Shape your mouth into an "O" shape and take short sips of air, all inhales, as if drinking the air, until full of breath, then hold. Roll your stomach in a small tight circle to the left, with a slight grind downward, ribs to hips. Halfway through your capacity to hold the breath, switch the direction of rotation to the right. When you can hold your breath no longer, straighten your spine and exhale slowly through your nose. Repeat once more.

2. Move to sitting on your heels, keeping your knees together. Relax your upper body forward, chest onto thighs and forehead to the floor. If you need to open your knees to make this accessible, that's fine. Your arms are relaxed down, in the posture commonly known as Child's Pose. Begin to move your hips from side to side, creating a U shape, with the bottom of the U centered over your heels and the upward sides of the U being created when you are left and right. Apply effort, imagining your hips are very heavy and dense. You'll feel the effort most in your lower abdomen and around your navel. Continue for 3 minutes, then rest for 5 minutes. ▷

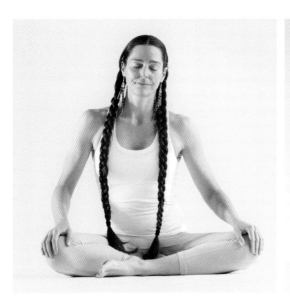 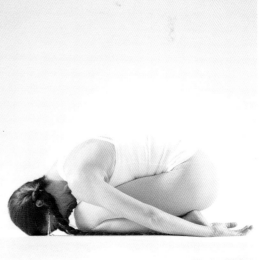

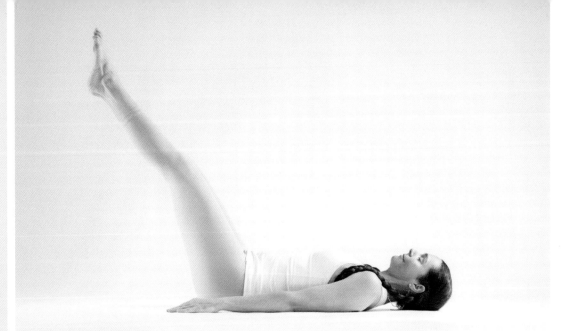

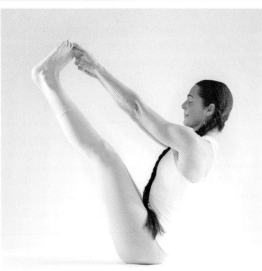

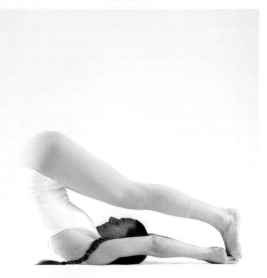

3. Lie down on your back. Point your toes, engage your legs, then lift your legs approximately 3 feet from the floor, keeping them locked together. You can place your hands under your lower back for support if needed. Do your best to hold this posture with long deep breathing (see page 5) for 2–3 minutes. Inhale, briefly hold the breath, then exhale and release your legs down.

4. Still on your back, bring both legs up to 90 degrees and catch your toes. Holding on to your toes, roll back and forth from the base of your spine to your neck. Continue rocking in this way for 2–3 minutes.

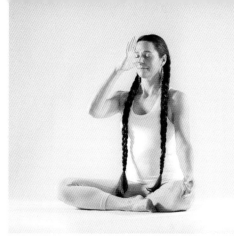
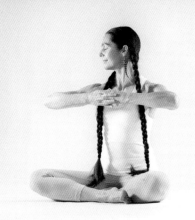
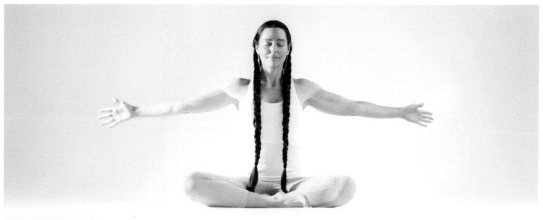

5. Move into Sukhasana. Here is one of the many variations possible in alternate nostril breathing: Bring your right thumb to your right nostril and seal the nostril. Inhale through your left nostril, then use your right index finger to seal your left nostril and release your thumb, exhaling through your right nostril. Continue this breath pattern for 3 minutes. Finish with a deep inhale through both nostrils.

6. Continue in Sukhasana. Place your hands into a Venus mudra by interlacing the fingers of each hand together. Bring the mudra up in front of your heart with your palms facing inward. Your arms should be in a loose circle. Inhale and turn just your head to the left; exhale and turn your head to the right. Do this for 2–3 minutes.

7. Still in Sukhasana, lift your arms straight out to the sides, from the shoulders, parallel to the ground with the palms down. Move both of your arms in backward circles for 1 minute. Then inhale deeply, holding the breath as you bend your elbows and touch your fingertips to your shoulders. Hold this breath and posture as long as is comfortable. See if you can feel the energy beginning to build in your body. Exhale, allowing the energy to flow through your entire body.

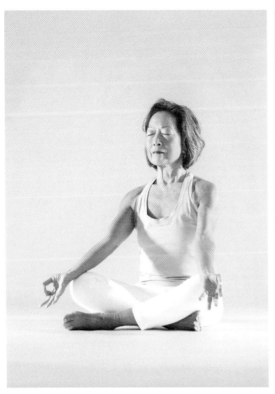 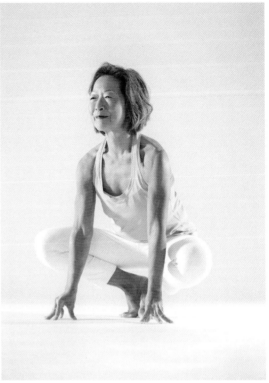

BODY BEAUTIFUL

This kriya has a special place in my heart. I confess to an inexplicable fondness for all variations of Frog Pose, which is said to open, free, and balance the energy of the sacral chakra, enhancing access to creative and sensual energy flow.

1. Seated in Sukhasana, rest your hands in any mudra. Bring attention to the breath, lengthening as well as deepening the breath. Meditate on the vitality and energy of the flow of breath for 3 minutes, with your eyes closed or holding a soft gaze. End with a deep inhale and hold the breath for a few seconds, then exhale and relax.

2. Go to a standing position for a powerful variation of Frog Pose: Fold forward from the waist, placing your fingertips on the floor, then squat down onto the balls of your feet with heels lifted and touching. Inhale, lifting your hips and dropping your head. Exhale, returning to the original posture. Your arms should not move; your fingertips provide balance and anchor. Do 10 repetitions of Frog, and on the tenth one, stay down and take three deep, complete breaths. On the third exhale, stay empty and squeeze mula bandha (root lock) for 10–20 seconds.

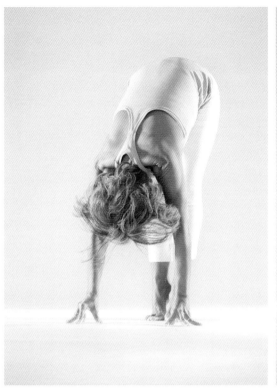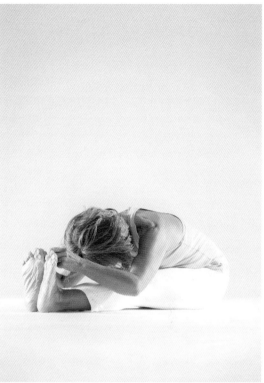

3. Repeat Frog Pose in this fashion 26 more times, again staying down on the last one. Take the three breaths and again apply mula bandha on the third exhale, sustaining the lock, void of breath for 10–20 seconds. See if you notice a flow of energy along the spine.

4. Relax down to a seated position, with your legs out in front. Fold forward, wrapping your big toes with the first two fingers of each hand, and apply gentle pressure with your thumb to the nail of your big toe (which stimulates the pituitary). Inhale, lengthen your spine, then exhale, folding forward, bringing your chest to your thighs and putting your head down, nose to knees. Hold this posture with long deep breathing (see page 5) for 3 minutes.

SEQUENCE TO RELIEVE PMS
or to Slow Down and Experience Gratitude

If you live in a body that doesn't bleed or experience PMS, explore this sequence during the waning of the moon. Waning energy is slowing, diminishing, and a wonderful time to experience gratitude for what is.

1. Sitting on your heels, rest your hands forward and extend your left leg straight back. Relax your torso forward, resting your head on the ground. Slide your arms back along your sides, palms up. Relax here for 3 minutes. Rise up, switch the legs, and repeat.

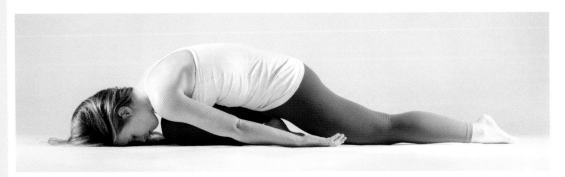

2. Return to sitting on your heels. Use your hands to gently massage all along your throat, from your collarbones to under your chin, for 2 minutes. Then, begin to massage your ears and earlobes with the palms of your hands for 2–3 minutes.

3. Still on your heels, place your hands in the Venus mudra at the small of your back. Inhale as you slowly twist your torso to the left, then exhale as you twist to the right, for 3 minutes. End with an inhale back at the center, consciously drawing the energy up your spine.

4. Relax down onto your back and bring your hands to your shoulders, fingers in front and thumbs on the back of your shoulders, elbows on the ground. Spread your legs comfortably wide. Tune in to all the muscles of your body and lift your upper body, bit by bit, as slowly as possible, until your torso is upright; then slowly fold forward from the waist until your nose is on the ground (or close to it). Hold this forward-fold version with long deep breathing (see page 5) for 3 minutes.

5. Return to lying on your back, in the same posture. This time, you'll repeat the lifting and folding, but the destination is nose to left knee, holding for 1 minute, concluding with 3 deep breaths. Return to your back and then repeat for the right knee.

▷

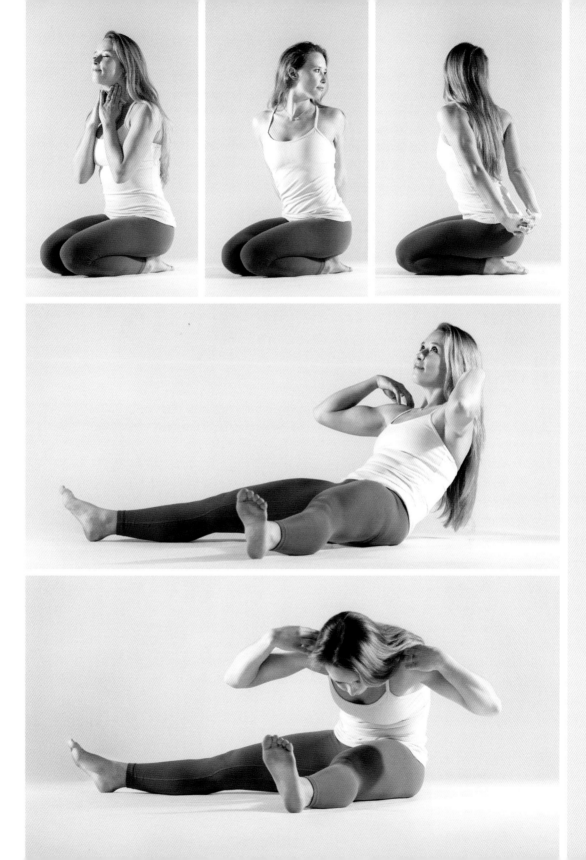

6. Come up from lying on your back and prepare for a little bit of wildness! Lower yourself onto your knees and elbows. Lift your hands and forearms so your elbows are supporting your upper body. Lift your head as well as your lower legs and begin to "walk" on your elbows and knees. Try and keep your feet pulled in to your thighs. You do not have to travel far but continue this walking motion for 3 minutes.

7. Completely relax on your back.

8. Sit upright and if accessible, take full Lotus Pose (each foot on the opposite thigh). If full Lotus is not possible, try half Lotus (one foot on one thigh). If neither of these postures is possible, take the Sukhasana posture with the tightest legs possible. Place your hands on the ground on either side of your hips. Push into your hands and swing your body forward. Bring your hands forward and again push into your arms to swing your body forward. Continue propelling your body forward with the strength of your arms for 3 minutes.

9. In the following dynamic version of Back Platform Pose, begin in a seated position, legs in front, feet hip-width apart. Place your hands on the ground behind you. Engage your legs and abdominals and lift your body up so you are balanced on your heels and hands. Begin "walking" in this pose. It's okay if your hips dip down, but try to keep your pelvis up and your body in a straight line. This takes significant effort—and again, you do not have to go far. Take little "steps" with your heels and hands for 1–2 minutes.

10. Relax onto your back into Shavasana. Completely and deeply let go. Consciously relax your entire body. Allow 10–15 minutes here to absorb and integrate the practice.

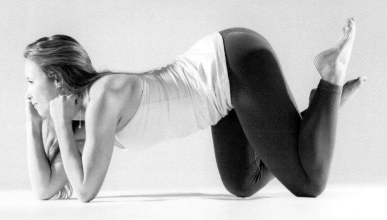

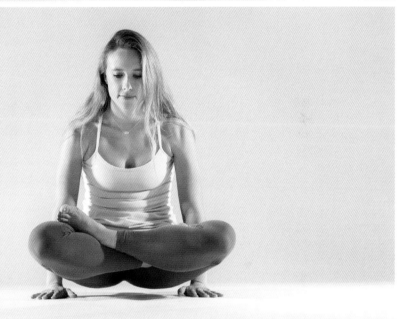

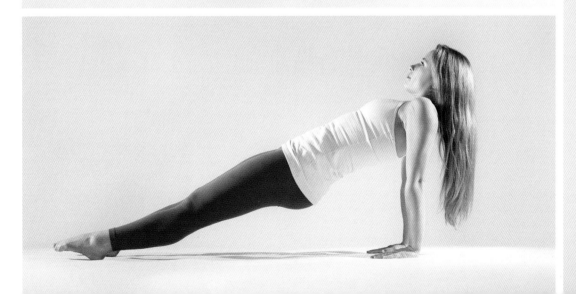

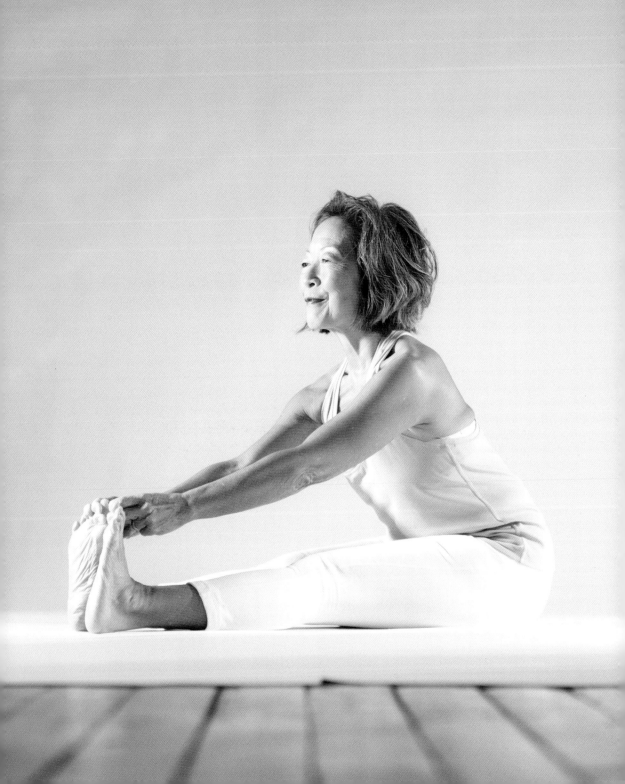

5

Practices for Any Time during the Lunar Cycle

THIS CHAPTER IS RICH with some of my favorite practices as well as some of the most powerful practices in the kundalini lexicon. Most days we are simply seeking movement that is beautiful and meaningful—a yoga practice for that day, rather than a practice that observes bleeding, pregnancy, or a moon phase.

The days that I practice yoga in the morning, right after my cup of tea, are always the best days. Beginning the day by moving the temple of body, honoring not only body but also spirit and mind, means that you have begun your day in *sadhana*, which in and of itself is a victory! The word *sadhana* simply means "practice," but it implies a committed daily and devoted practice. The kundalini tradition has additional connotations regarding sadhana: in kundalini practice, sadhana often takes place before the sun rises and includes devotional readings and mantra chanting as well as asana and kriya.

When I was young and new to yoga, full of enthusiasm and little experience, I would set myself impossible sadhana goals. Arising at 3:30 a.m. and beginning lengthy and complicated practices that would take me until sunrise was not sustainable over the long run. If you are not yet a dedicated practitioner, I would encourage you to simply set the intention of some form of practice every day. Let your goal be consistency in showing up on your mat. Some days might be twenty minutes, some days an hour, some days a bit of reading and a few postures. If you don't make it to your mat in the morning, all is not lost—hopefully you can get to some practice time later in the day. I do find that practice first results in a better day, and there is just ease in knowing you have done your sadhana versus having it wait for you.

A goal of consistency is what will serve you in the long run. It can be helpful to choose a specific practice or kriya and stick with that practice for 40 days. It is true that there is a natural rhythm to our habits in body and mind, and 40 days of consistent practice enables us to experience the effects of the kriya and understand the practice in a clearer light. To break the habit of not practicing every day, you practice for 40 days in a row. To establish the new habit in action, in the subconscious, you commit to 90 days. To confirm the new consciousness and effects of the practice more permanently, you practice for 120 days. To master the practice and be able to call upon the gift of the practice in any challenge, a thousand-day sadhana is prescribed. Over the course of thirty-plus years, I've done many 40-, 90-, and 120-day practices and can vouch for the rewards of a dedicated practice. As I write this book, I am approaching the completion of my first thousand-day sadhana, and the beauty of a daily practice that spans almost three years is profound. My practice has become almost a sutra of sorts—a thread of consciousness and continuity that overrides and outlives the trials and tribulations of any given period (see sidebar).

The word *yoga* comes from the Sanskrit root *yuj*, meaning "to yoke," which also means "to join" or "to unite": as you practice, keep in mind that the intention in yoga is not to carve our bodies to look a certain way or to achieve certain postures but rather to yoke all aspects of our being in order to awaken into our wisest, kindest, truest selves. To separate yoga from this fullness, to reduce it to simply exercise, is to miss the point. While it is true that yoga can absolutely result in a stronger, fitter body and better health, I would encourage you to seek out another modality (weights, cardio, swimming, or running, for example) if your motivation for practicing yoga is simply physical. That said, in no way is it meant to diminish the goals of physical fitness! On the contrary, caring for our bodies is an important part of the yogic path—but it is just one aspect of the practice. Stepping onto a yoga mat is an agreement to living yoga off of the mat as well. To embark upon the path of yoga is ultimately to agree to the great and universal vows of the beginning path and to commit to embodying the teachings, to the best of your ability, in every moment, with every breath. The great and universal vows of the beginning path of yoga are collectively known as "the eight-limbed path" and are covered in chapter 10, "Yoga Is a Call to Action."

It is valuable to examine and occasionally reexamine our goals from time to time. Over many years of working with students, especially those who identify as women, I've come to understand that sometimes our desire for our bodies to look or feel a certain way is not linked to health—and worse, isn't really an organic desire in our own hearts. The pressure on the female body to look a certain way is intense,

SUTRA

Sutra is a Sanskrit word that translates to "thread" or "string" but can also refer to a condensed rule or scripture. A sutra is a teaching that is purposely compressed and dense with meaning and layer. Sutras are meant to be unwoven and expounded upon with a teacher or in communion with other learners. The thread of a sutra invites following or pursuing it to a fuller meaning and message. The thread-like nature of sutras also lends them to being woven with other sutras for a larger tapestry or fabric of teachings. The most well-known example of this would be Patanjali's Yoga Sutras.

relentless, unrealistic, and ultimately not driven by anyone or anything that has your best interest in mind. All too often, the media message around the feminine body is driven by capitalism, motivated by control and the acquisition of consumers. Quite often, it boils down to selling an unachievable ideal that results in women buying all sorts of things in a never-ending quest to achieve the impossible, while also distracting us from the things that truly need our attention. The psychology of marketing has become ever smarter and slicker and is now insidious.

Somewhat ironically, these same marketing strategies and impossible glossy images have also permeated the yoga industry. Nonetheless, the committed practice of yoga will deliver us to the understanding that the treasure we seek is within us, not available for purchase outside of us. As much as yoga is about our relationship with the world, it is also about our relationship with ourselves. It is one of my deepest wishes that we love our bodies deeply, that we befriend our bodies, and that the requests we make of our bodies are organized around health. Health is more what you feel than what you see: Having a healthy heart. Nourishing yourself with whole foods. Getting enough rest. Moving, sweating, laughing, connecting. Finding purpose in life and work and relationship. Finding a way to make our little patch of earth a place where all life is cared for and sustained with love.

Yoga is and has always been a spiritual practice. In moving our bodies through shapes, flows, asana, with breath and mindfulness, we experience the full and total union with our truest, deepest self—and in so doing, we create that connection to everything else. Yoga has the potential to heal our bodies, our minds, our spirits. When we choose how we wish to practice for the day, we can and should bring an understanding of what we wish to move and what might need extra care in our bodies. Sometimes it can be just as simple as wishing to express gratitude to the moon and the sun, or to the breath. Sometimes it can be understanding that we really need something restorative and relaxing. It might seem like a paradox, but I've found that the more mindfulness I can bring to my practice, coupled with less focus on "rules" or "goals," the more fulfilling the practices turn out to be. Don't be afraid to come to your mat with no plan beyond befriending your body and spending time with yourself. Some of my favorite practices of all time have consisted of just moving on my mat to music or chants that are meaningful to me. Trust the innate wisdom of your body, of your heart, and of your soul.

Deeply listening to ourselves is one way to choose our practice. Another way to choose is to consider the Vedic wisdom embodied in Ayurveda, which tells us that three *doshas*, or types of energy, are at play within each of us: *kapha*, which is the energy of earth and water; *pitta*, the energy of fire and water; and *vata*, the energy of air and ether. The interplay of the doshas within us is both an expression of our basic nature and a determining force of our physical constitution. Ayurveda is an incredibly complex and nuanced science as well as being a philosophy. I asked Shala Worsley, an Ayurvedically influenced yoga teacher and friend, if it would be possible to simplify the concepts a bit for dosha-informed practice, and she created these wonderful guidelines to practice for you:

○ ○ ○ ○ ○

Doshas: Identifying, Balancing, and Practice

1. Identify your *prakriti*, which is your underlying constitutional type, and practice yoga in a way that pacifies that dosha. To identify your dosha you can take online dosha quizzes, but those can be potentially misleading. The best way to identify your prakriti is to consult with an Ayurvedic professional.

2. Identify your *vikriti*, which is your current dosha imbalance. Practice yoga in a way that soothes the dosha you have identified as out of balance until balance has been restored.

Dosha-Informed Practice

Feeling frazzled, spacey, exhausted, or anxious? Pacify vata. Do practices that help you get grounded, warm, and steady; practice with regularity.

Feeling driven, hyper-focused, irritable, or impatient? Pacify pitta. Do yoga that helps you slow down, chill out, be playful, and space out.

Feeling sluggish, heavy, lethargic, or withdrawn? Pacify kapha. Do yoga that helps you get sweaty; challenge yourself, change positions often, and vary your routines frequently.

If this approach resonates with you, consider learning more about Ayurveda and ways to sync your yoga practice to the rhythms of nature.

○ ○ ◯ ○ ○

I've included six specific practices for your consideration, on any given day—actually, seven practices if you take my advice to just free flow to music sometimes.

For Radiance, Vitality, and Grace is an occasional must for those who identify as living in a lunar body! With this practice, which includes Camel Pose, Shoulderstand, Archer Pose, Bow Pose, and Stretch Pose, you are moving through some of the primary poses for a woman's body. While I've listed a number of postures that many will already be familiar with, there are detailed descriptions as well as pictures for those readers who are novice practitioners. One of the things that I especially appreciate about this sequence is that it is open-ended—you can assign the times for each posture based on the amount of time that you have to spend doing your practice on any given day. You can even skip poses and change up the breath, depending on the day. This is a great template as well for just choosing portions of the sequence to complement some free or structured flow movements.

I've included the most basic **Sun Salutation (Surya Namaskar)** here—I am a huge fan of salutations in general and very rarely does a day slip by that I don't do at least a few salutations. Sun greetings are a great warm-up before a meditation or shorter kriya. I love the way the basic Sun Salutation allows me the opportunity to feel gratitude for the sun as well as to stay strong and flexible. Once you feel comfortable with this basic salutation, I encourage embellishing it! Play with moving from Downward Facing Dog (Adho Mukha Svanasana) to one of the Warrior Poses or a balance pose and then flow back to Downward Facing Dog and repeat on the other side. This salutation is foundational, at the heart of *vinyasa*, a Sanskrit word rich with meaning that benefits from context. The root of this word, *nyasa*, means "to place," and the *vi* prefix translates to "in a special way." Here, in this context, it is shorthand for linking the breath with flowing movement, allowing the intelligence of breath and intuition to guide you into shapes and transitions that your body is craving. In other contexts, *vinyasa* can refer to the specific steps to take for a desired outcome or a specific style of yoga.

The **Moon Salutation (Chandra Namaskar)** is, hands down, my absolute favorite practice in the universe! Like the sun greetings, moon greetings have multiple versions. The Moon Salutation that I've included here is the one that has always spoken most deeply to my heart and felt the most in tune and rhythm with the moon and all her phases. I tend to save Moon Salutations for full moon and new moon days, but you can do them anytime you like! Classic yoga, as codified by Patanjali, has always emphasized that pranayama (our breath) is the priority in our practice. What this means is that we never sacrifice our breath for a posture; rather, if there is a sacrifice to be made, it is letting go of the posture before compromising our breath. And yet—the reality of yoga and our efforts! I know that I have often sacrificed my breath in the execution of a posture, especially the more difficult asanas.

When we come to the **Moon Salutation** and the variations, it feels like coming home to a sweet reprieve. Here, we just breathe. We do not move on the breath, nor do we control or count the breath. We simply flow, breathing, through the salutation. When we find ourselves in the more constricted postures, if our breath becomes shorter and somewhat more constricted, we allow that. There is a harmony here, in these salutations. If your body seeks a fuller, more expansive breath as you fold forward from the Star Pose (Tarasana) then you embrace and allow that. Moon Salutations are a witnessing of how the shape of our bodies organically influences our breath. I find that so refreshing and it makes a lovely break from more solar executions of yoga.

While I cannot recall the original source of my learning of this version, I believe that it was tantric sourced. Yoga has taken two very different paths with regard to philosophy around moon days. Think of Ashtanga—as noted in chapter 4, this is a practice that advocates rest on the moon days. The lineages that are sourced from the tantric stream do not break from practice on moon days, but instead they invoke and honor the moon on those days.

The last three practices that I have included in this chapter—**Sat Kriya**, **Kirtan Kriya**, and **Sodharshan Chakra Kriyas**—are widely considered to be not only the most powerful and transforming practices of kundalini yoga but also the triad of practices that will hold and steer us through anything.

Sat Kriya can be translated to "true complete action." The word *kriya*, as already discussed, means "action," yet it also implies that the action is complete. *Sat* is interpreted variously as "true" or "truth." This little practice is considered complete in and of itself. If you are an experienced yoga practitioner, there is a good chance that you are already familiar with **Sat Kriya**; although it is a complete practice, it is also often the jewel within a larger kriya as well. The benefits we receive when we practice **Sat Kriya** are many, including a mild massage of our internal organs, enhanced circulation (both physically and energetically) throughout our bodies, a strengthening of our entire sexual system, and a boosting and balancing effect on the flow of kundalini energy in our bodies. When the flow of our kundalini energy is unimpeded and our bodies are healthy, we experience creative inspiration as well as healing.

Kirtan Kriya is one of the most beautiful and influential meditations I have ever encountered! It is taught that this one practice completely balances our minds as well as our psyche. The word *kirtan* is Sanskrit for "song" or "praise," and here, our action is complete with songs or chants of praise. **Kirtan Kriya** enhances longevity, health, and well-being. While this practice is embedded deep, through source and lineage in the kundalini tradition, the last few decades have seen this meditation become a global practice, far outside of the realm of kundalini yoga. Numerous research studies (some cited by the authors in the resources section of this book) have confirmed that this meditation improves memory and cognitive performance, reduces the experience of stress as well as depression, and is thought to improve overall brain chemistry. The research suggests that it works to ward off the cognitive decline that can be a part of the aging process: one exciting study done at UCLA indicated that regular practice actually reverses the shrinking of telomeres—the ends of DNA strands that protect our chromosomes. As we age, our telomeres inevitably shrink to some degree, but people with conditions such as dementia or Alzheimer's disease often have accelerated withering of telomeres. Practicing **Kirtan Kriya** on a regular basis can not only delay the aging of the brain, it can also reverse it! A variation of **Kirtan Kriya** that balances the moon centers of our bodies is also provided at the end.

Sodharshan Chakra Kriya is considered to be one of the simplest as well as, paradoxically, one of the most difficult meditations to practice. The instructions for practice are straightforward enough, yet the level of control at the navel center is demanding. The word *darshan* is derived from the Sanskrit word *darsana*, which means "sight" or "vision." *Sodharshan* means "pure sight or pure vision," and combined with the words *chakra* (energy wheel) and *kriya*, the name conveys that this meditation is one that brings us the complete experience of pure and large vision through wheels of energy. Another way to understand what happens when we practice this kriya is to consider that we are embarking on a journey that will transform us and support us on our highest path. Within the kundalini tradition, this is considered the highest kriya of all, one that will not only cleanse our subconscious but also eliminate any darkness that impedes our fulfillment.

FOR RADIANCE, VITALITY, AND GRACE

1. Begin sitting on your heels—some traditions call this seated Thunderbolt Pose (Vajrasana) and the kundalini tradition refers to it as Rock Pose. Inhale as you flex your spine forward, then exhale flexing backward until your spine feels flexible and awake. Come back to center and meditate at the brow point with long deep breathing (see page 5) for 2 minutes.

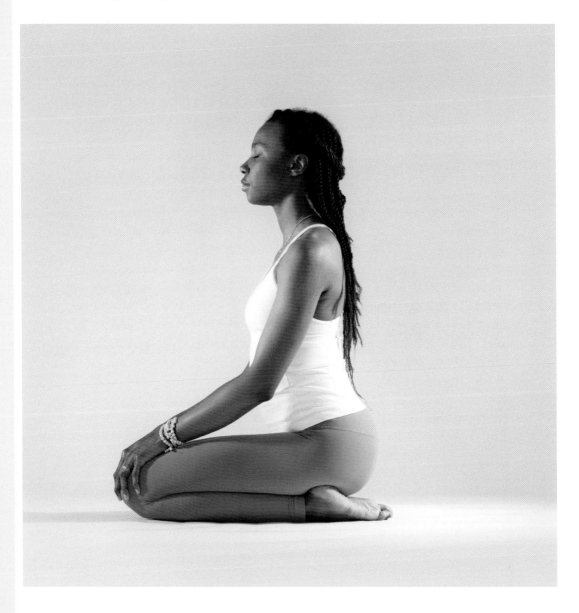

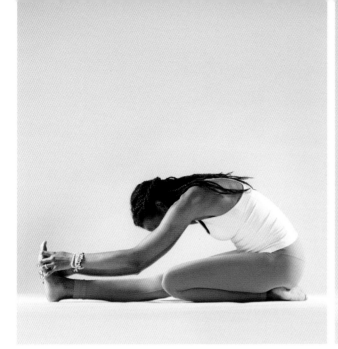
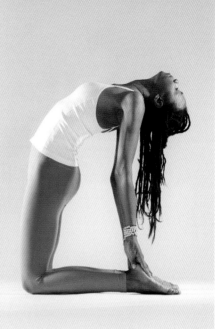

2. Extend your left leg forward, continuing to sit on your right heel. Hold your toes and draw your heart toward your left knee. You can do breath of fire (page 5) or long deep breathing (page 5) for 2–3 minutes, then switch sides and repeat.

3. Come up on your knees, with knees hip-width apart. Reach back for your heels, releasing your head back while also bringing your hips forward and lifting your sternum high—this is Camel Pose. If this pose feels like too much sensation in your low back, you can modify it by bringing the palms to the backs of your thighs. Choose your breath and time here.

4. Shoulderstand. The key with this posture is not to turn your head but to gaze steadily at the ceiling—this is to protect your neck. Tuck your knees in toward your chest and then unfold, bringing your legs up and slightly over your head while drawing your arms in and placing your hands under your hips for support. The weight of your body is on your shoulders but also your upper arms, through the support of your hips with your hands. It is less important to get perfectly straight and more important to stay mindful. If your chest comes into your chin, that is fine and actually beneficial for the thyroid gland. Do a long deep breathing pattern here (page 5), continuing for 1–2 minutes.

▷

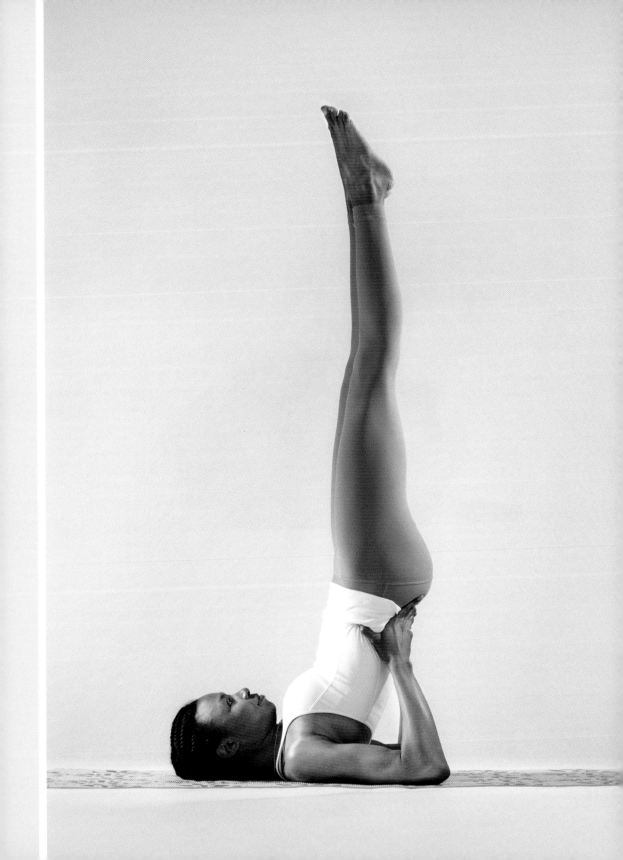

5. Come to a standing position and step your left leg forward, bending your knee over your ankle, right leg straight back, right foot turned slightly in. Lift your left arm straight in front and imagine you are holding a heavy archer's bow. Draw the string back with your right arm. Create a muscular tension in both arms: one holding the heavy bow, the other drawing back a heavy and resistant string. Hold with your choice of breath for 2–3 minutes, then switch and do the other side.

6. Return to seated Thunderbolt (or Rock) Pose, then release your chest forward onto your thighs, head on the ground, arms relaxed back for Child's Pose. Really let go and feel supported and relaxed for 1–2 minutes. ▷

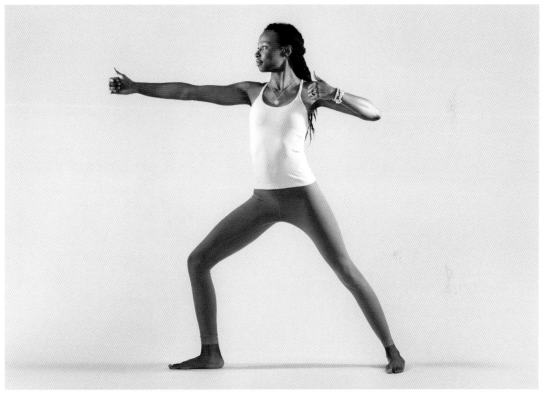

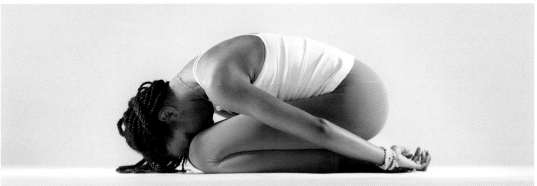

7. Move to lying on your stomach, initially lengthening the torso, then bend your knees and catch your ankles. Arching your back, lift your head, chest, and legs up—this is Bow Pose. Hold with your choice of breath for 2–3 minutes.

8. Relax down onto your stomach and move into a variation of Locust Pose by placing gently held fists under your hips and above the tops of your legs. The palm side of your fists is turned upward, into the body. Relax your head onto your chin and inhale, lifting both legs up in the air. Hold with your breath choice for as long as possible.

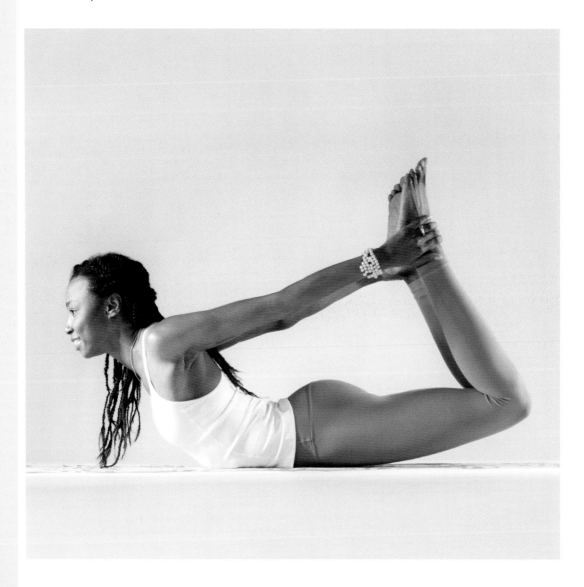

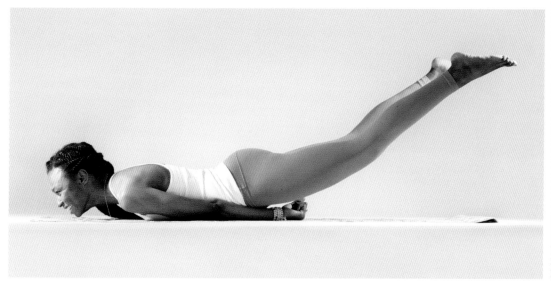

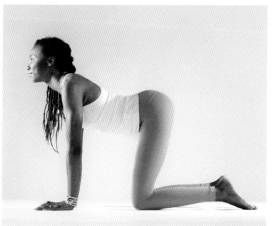
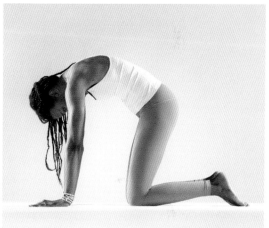

9. Move into a table shape with hands below the shoulders and knees beneath the hips. From here, tilt the top of the pelvis toward the floor, which also results in the base of the pelvis lifting toward the sky. Let your belly drop toward the floor, becoming sway-backed. The head is lifted, and the dhristi, or gaze, is skyward. This is Cow Pose. Hold this position with long deep breathing (page 5) for 2–3 minutes.

10. Return to the more neutral table shape and then tuck your entire pelvis toward your navel. Release your head toward the earth and arch your spine upward like a cat. And lo and behold, you are now in Cat Pose. Hold this position for the same amount of time as you held Cow Pose.

▷

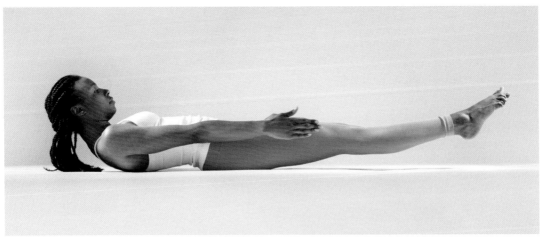

11. Lie down on your back. Lift and tuck your pelvis slightly and then rerelease your low back down to the floor (this can be helpful to really access your core abdominal muscles). Lift your feet, toes pointed and heels together, 6 inches off the floor. Lift your head off the floor and gaze at your feet while also lifting your arms up, alongside your body with the palms facing each other. Hold this Stretch Pose with a breath of fire (page 5) for 1–3 minutes. If this is too challenging, slide your hands under your low back for extra support and try again.

12. Relax on your back for as long as you like.

13. End with **Sat Kriya** (page 86) for 3–5 minutes.

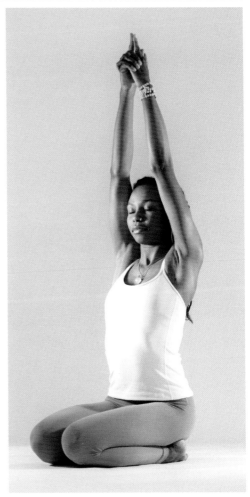

SUN SALUTATION (SURYA NAMASKAR)

1. Step to the top of your mat and place your feet inside the outer line of your hips, parallel to each other. Your arms are relaxed down by your sides. This is Mountain Pose, or Tadasana. Allow yourself to feel strong and grounded here.

2. Inhale, sweeping your arms up and over your head.

3. Exhale, folding fully forward and placing your palms on the floor if possible.

▷

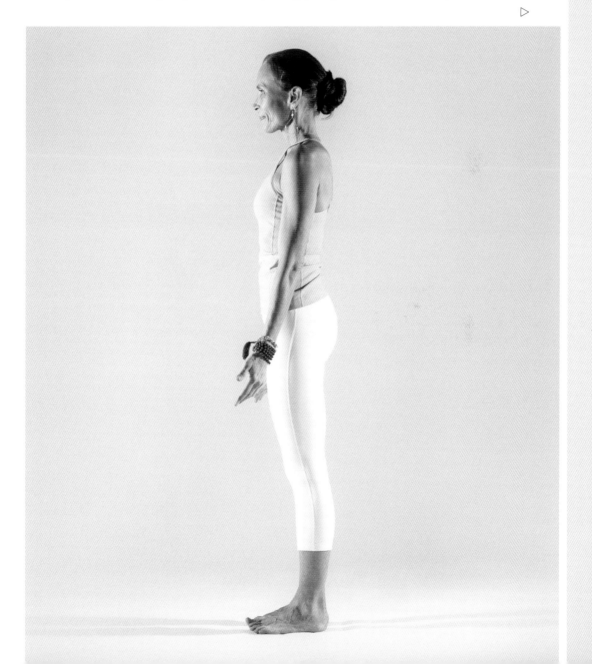

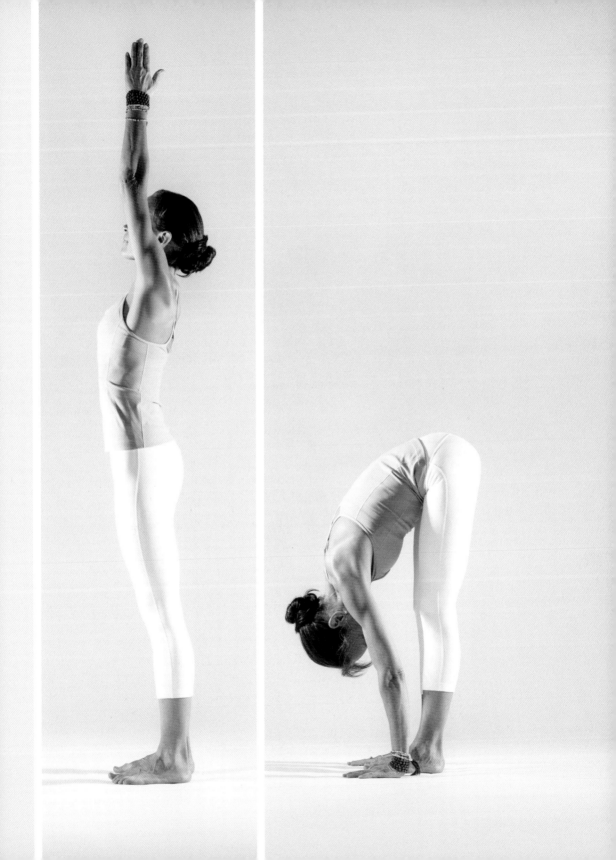

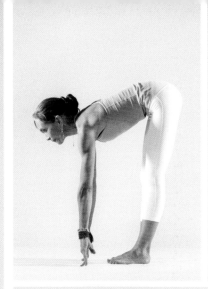
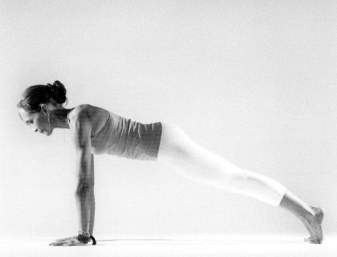
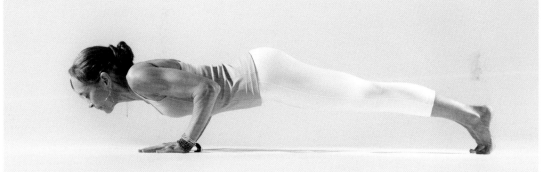

4. Inhale as you lift your head and torso halfway up, allow the hands to organically follow the energy of the lift, coming up to the fingertips. Still on the inhale, having reached halfway up, you'll release the tension a bit so you can place your hands on your mat, underneath the shoulders.

5. Without releasing your inhale, step or hop back to a high Plank; the hands stay under the shoulders, arms straight. The body is straight (like a plank of wood) and the balls of the feet are the only other contact with the mat. (In the Ashtanga lineage and many "power flow" forms, you would jump directly back to Four-Limbed Staff Pose, or Chaturanga Dandasana).

6. From this high Plank position, exhale down to Chaturanga Dandasana, which is the posture shown in the photo, or you can modify this step and take your body all the way down to the floor, which is much less strenuous and fits in to the sequence flow beautifully. Another option is to lower the knees to your mat and take the shape of chaturanga with just the upper body. Ultimately, the shape you take in this step has everything to do with the shape you wish to take in the next step.

▷

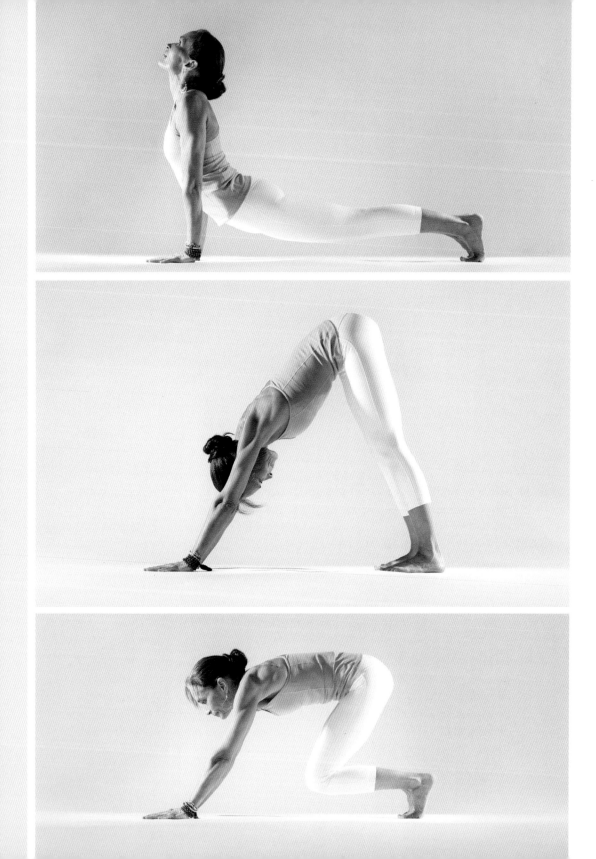

7. Inhale to Upward Facing Dog or Cobra. Upward Facing Dog is shown in the photo and is predicated on moving from Chaturanga. Pushing into the balls of your feet, glide forward, lifting the torso, dropping the hips, and moving onto the tops of your feet. Or, if you are moving from having released the front body to the floor, bring your heels together, press lightly into your hands, and use your back muscles to lift your chest and head up.

8. Releasing the tension of either Upward Facing Dog or Cobra, take your exhale as you lift your hips skyward and create a triangle shape with your body. This is Downward Facing Dog and widely considered to be a "rest pose." The head and neck are relaxed. (It is traditional to take 5 deep and complete breaths here and find the resting energy in this posture).

9. After the last exhale, still void of breath, lift your gaze to your hands and step or hop your feet to your hands.

10. Inhale, halfway up, as in step 4.

11. Exhale, folding down, as in step 3.

12. Inhale, rising to standing and sweeping your arms fully up and over your head, as in step 2.

13. Exhale, bringing your hands to your heart (in Anjali mudra) or down to your sides (Mountain Pose).

You can do as many Sun Salutations as you like. These can be a great way to warm up before another practice, be a transition between practices, or serve as your entire practice on some days!

I'd like to offer some further commentary for any readers that might be new to Sun Salutations. As mentioned in the instructional steps, the photos accompanying this **Sun Salutation** demonstrate moving from high Plank Pose to Chaturanga Dandasana. To do this, you'll want to draw your shoulder blades slightly together and down the back while still in high Plank. Keep your arms close to your body as you lower to Chaturanga. If this feels too intense or if you need to build upper body strength a bit before attempting, lower your knees to the floor from high Plank and work on keeping your spine straight as you continue to the floor. As mentioned during the steps, you can also simply lower directly and entirely to the floor. From here, it is more somatically congruent to take Cobra rather than Upward Facing Dog. You always have the option to substitute Cobra for Up Dog even if it hasn't been made explicit. My opinion is that Upward Facing Dog really does not offer greater benefit than Cobra beyond being a physically logical move from Chaturanga.

MOON SALUTATION (CHANDRA NAMASKAR)

Enjoy the flow of breath in response to the posture. See if you can let your body lead you in how long you stay in each shape and when you transition.

1. Step to the middle of your mat. This is the "home" of moon (in contrast to standing at the top of the mat when practicing **Sun Salutation**). Bring the feet together, touching, and lift the hands to the heart in Anjali mudra.

2. Sweep your arms up over your head and bringing your palms together, stretch your spine up.

3. Drop over to your left side, keeping your knees, hips, shoulders, and head aligned. This posture is known as Upward Salute Side Bend, or Parsva Urdhva Hastasana.

4. Return to the center, again stretching your spine up.

5. Drop over to your right side, replicating the posture of step 3, taking Upward Salute Side Bend on the other side.

6. Return to center, stretching up.

7. Gently engage your gluteus muscles, bring your pelvis slightly forward, and lift your sternum skyward as you drop back. It might just be looking at the ceiling or it could be a deeper drop back, depending upon your body. There is no need to push. Instead, let your body reveal to you the depth of the arch and drop that can be given. This is a version of Standing Backbend, or Anuvittasana.

▷

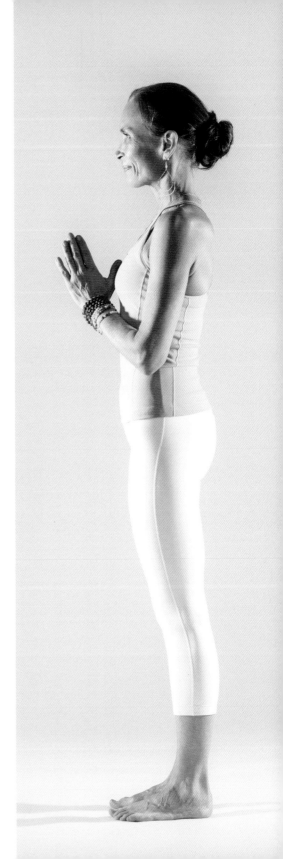

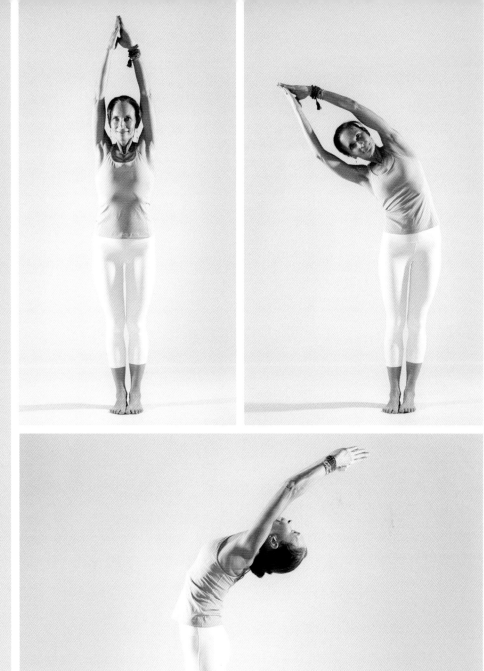

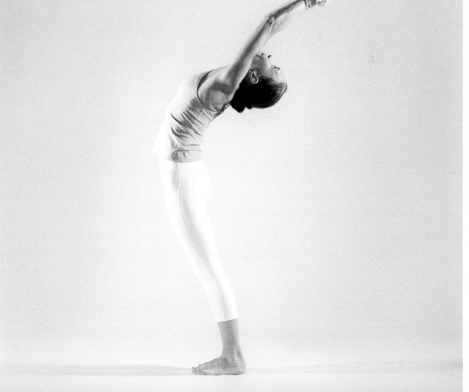

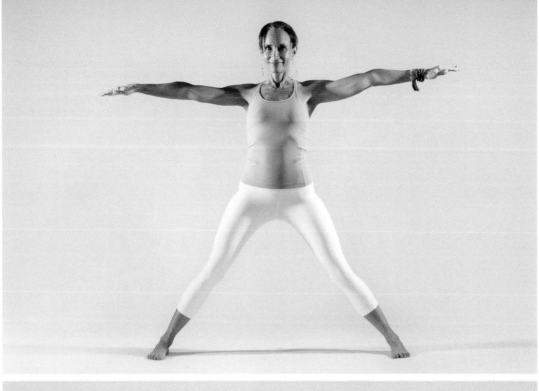

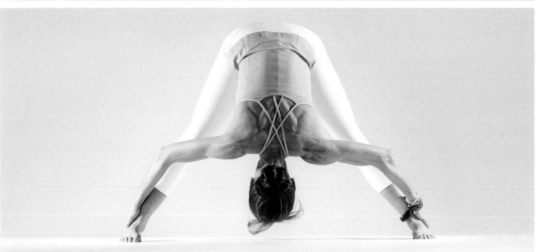

8. Step to a wide straddle, feet parallel to each other and your arms extended to the sides, palms down. Relax your shoulders here. This is the Star Pose, or Tarasana.

9. Stretching your spine forward, keeping your arms out, fold yourself forward. You have several options you could choose to pursue in the fold. You can grasp opposite elbows and allow yourself to hang, or you could place your palms on the floor, or you could pursue a deeper fold by holding the outside of your ankles and engaging a bit of arm leverage to pull yourself in deeper.

10. Release the position you have taken with your arms or hands and let your arms float back out to your sides; rise up slowly, bringing your arms overhead, palms touching. Reduce the width of your stance by "heel-toeing" your feet together twice.

11. Keeping your palms together and arms up, step your left foot forward, turn your torso to the left, and shift so that your left foot is straight forward; angle your right foot forward as well. Take the time to adjust your hips square to the top of your mat. If you have tight hips, this can be achieved by creating a little more distance in the horizontal width of your stance, as if sending the outer sides of your feet away from the center of your mat.

12. Stretch your spine up and then fold forward, finding the most resonant way to be in this shape. You can rest your hands on your shins, rest your hands to the floor on either side of your feet, or keep your palms together, letting your fingertips graze the ground.

13. Ground your feet, strengthen your legs, and slowly rise back up in the reverse of the way you folded down, ultimately with arms overhead, palms together.   ▷

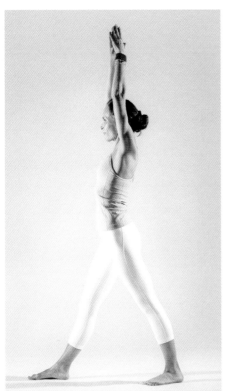 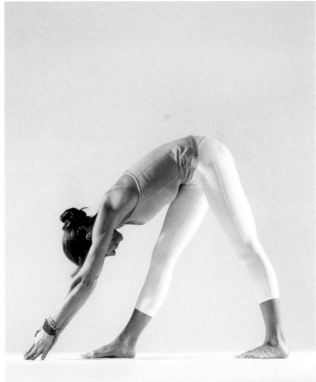

14. Pivot your feet back to the center.

15. Pivot to the right, with your right foot forward, taking the time to align your pelvis and torso forward, as in step 11.

16. Repeat the movements as instructed in step 12 but now to the right.

17. Repeat step 13.

18. Repeat step 14.

19. Step or hop your feet together.

20. Fold forward to the earth, and again you can choose between options: finding opposite elbows and hanging, placing your hands on the earth, or reaching behind your feet for a deeper fold.

21. Bringing your hands back together, rise back up with your arms overhead.

22. Step with your left foot to the top of mat, sending your right leg back for a deep but high lunge (back leg lifted versus knee down), up on the ball of your right foot. This posture is variously known as Vanarasana or Banarasana, but I've only

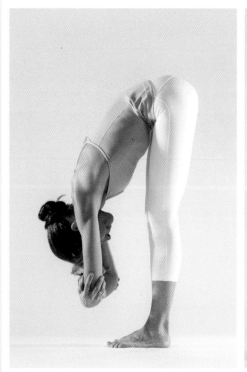
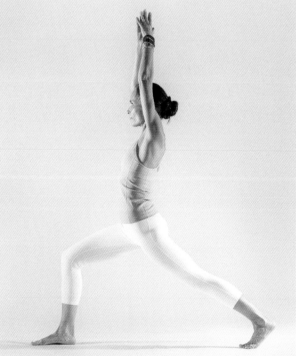

ever heard teachers say "high lunge." The arms are lifted here and there is less stability than a Warrior version with the back heel down. You could choose to stay here and skip the next pose or continue to step 23.

23. From high lunge, with the arms lifted, drop your upper body back, creating the shape of a crescent moon from the heels up the arch of the back to the fingertips. This posture is called Crescent Moon, or Ashta Chandrasana. The translation would be "eighth of the moon."

24. Return to the lunge position and float your fingers down to frame your front foot.

25. Bring your back leg forward, go high on your toes, sit down on your heels, and arch your spine, tucking into a posture that can represent the full or new moon. Relax your head here.

26. Lift your gaze and send your left leg back, moving into a deep high lunge on the other side, up on the ball of your back foot—as in step 22 but now on the other side.

27. Again here, you can choose to take Crescent Moon Pose or skip to the next posture.

▷

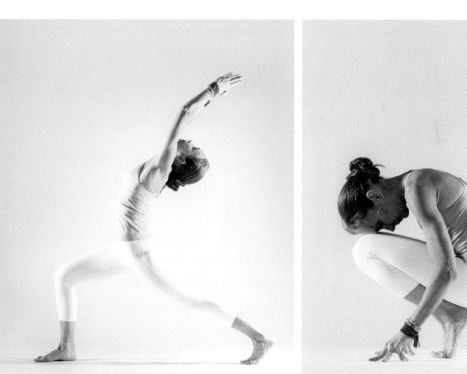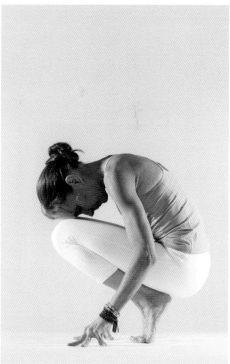

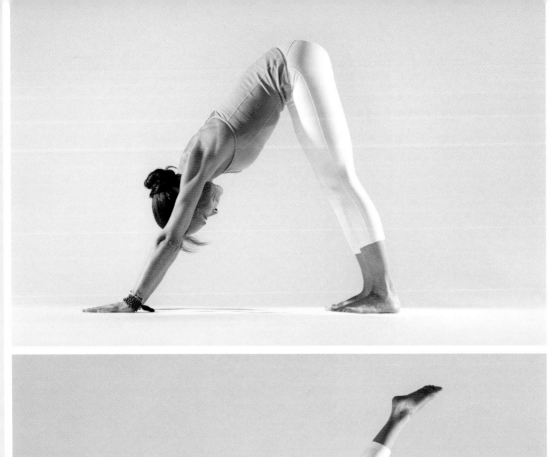

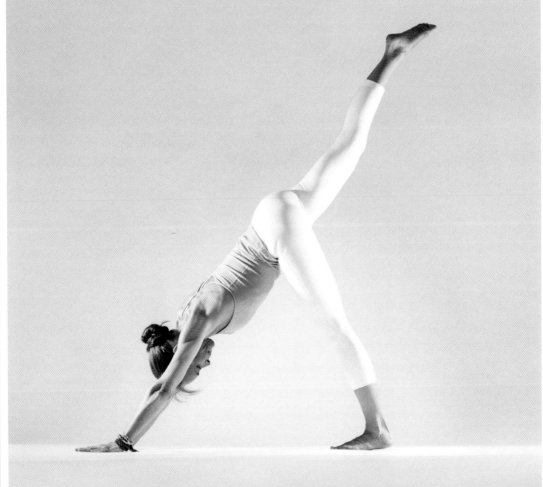

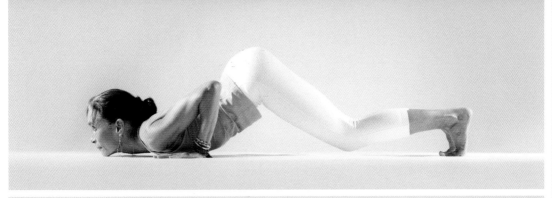

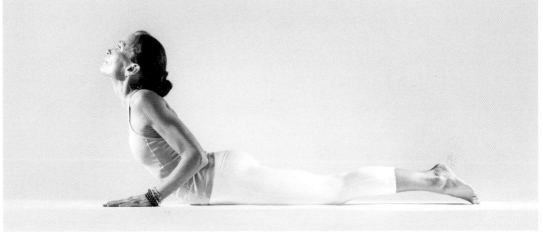

28. Release your hands down to frame your front foot, shoulder-width apart, and step back to Downward Facing Dog.

29. Lift your left leg up, ideally to where the line of the leg continues the line of the spine.

30. Release your left leg down, then raise your right leg up, and eventually back down, returning to Downward Facing Dog.

31. Shift your shoulders over your hands, bend your knees and hover; if this feels like too much, release your knees to your mat.

32. Bring first your chin, then your chest, then the rest of your body down to your mat. This posture is a form of *pranam* meaning "to bend" or "to bow to." In this salutation, each step, each posture is a pranam to the moon.

33. Bring your heels together, and gently engage the muscles of the legs and lift the torso up into Cobra Pose.

34. Release Cobra Pose while simultaneously coiling your body back.

▷

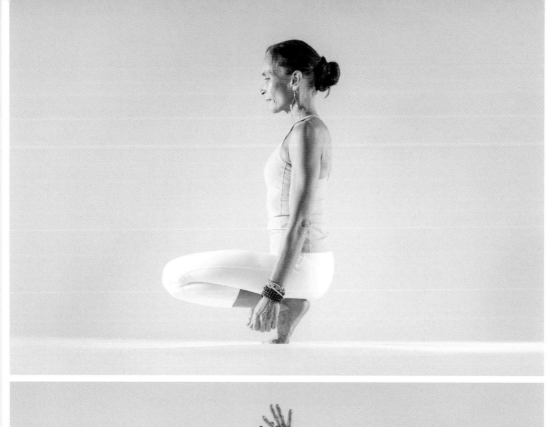

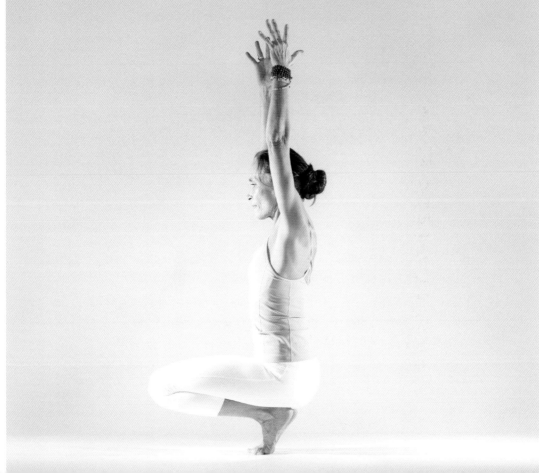

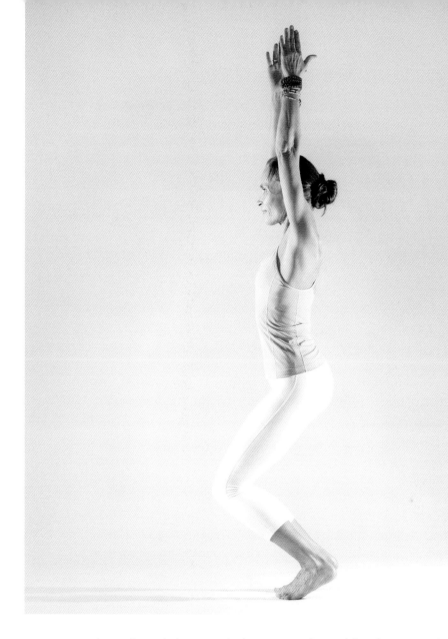

35. Release the coiled tension by hopping to the middle of your mat, landing on the balls of your feet and toes. Find your balance on your toes.

36. Lift your arms overhead with palms facing each other, and pause for a moment here, continuing to balance. Then squeeze your thighs together, and rise on your toes back to standing.

37. Release your hands down to your heart as your heels come down. Release your arms to the sides.

SAT KRIYA

Begin this kriya sitting on your heels in Rock Pose. You can sit up on a yoga block or cushion if the heel-sitting posture is uncomfortable; as with anything, practice will make the posture more accessible.

Interlace your fingers and release your index fingers upward, locking the mudra with your left thumb if you would like to emphasize moon energy or with your right thumb to emphasize sun energy. Lift your arms overhead, with your upper arms aligning with your ears. Set your spine tall and imagine a spine as strong and unyielding as a wall; don't allow yourself to bend or buckle once you begin.

Chant SAT ("truth" or "true") as you pull your navel in and up, also inhaling. Chant NAM as you release your navel and exhale. You are striving for a constant and steady rhythm of about 7 or 8 pulls per 10 seconds: too fast and it is difficult to get a good contraction at the navel; too slow and the breath becomes challenging to regulate. Let the vibration of SAT be the vibration of effort at the navel point. Allow the vibration of NAM to be focused at the brow point and felt as relaxing.

Practice for 3–31 minutes. Build the length of time you practice slowly.

To end the kriya, inhale and squeeze the energy, as well as your muscles (gently), from the base of the spine up to base of the neck. Hold the breath and energy for a few seconds as you focus and imagine the energy ascending to a point above the head. Exhale completely, relaxing the muscles but maintaining the posture. Inhale deeply, exhale completely, and squeeze maha bandha—the great lock. Keep breath out, with the lock held for 10 or so seconds. Then release maha bandha and tension. Inhale and relax.

Sat Kriya is considered a complete practice. It is traditional to relax for a time equal to the amount of time you spent doing **Sat Kriya** if this is your entire practice. If **Sat Kriya** is part of another kriya, follow the guidelines for relaxation indicated in the kriya.

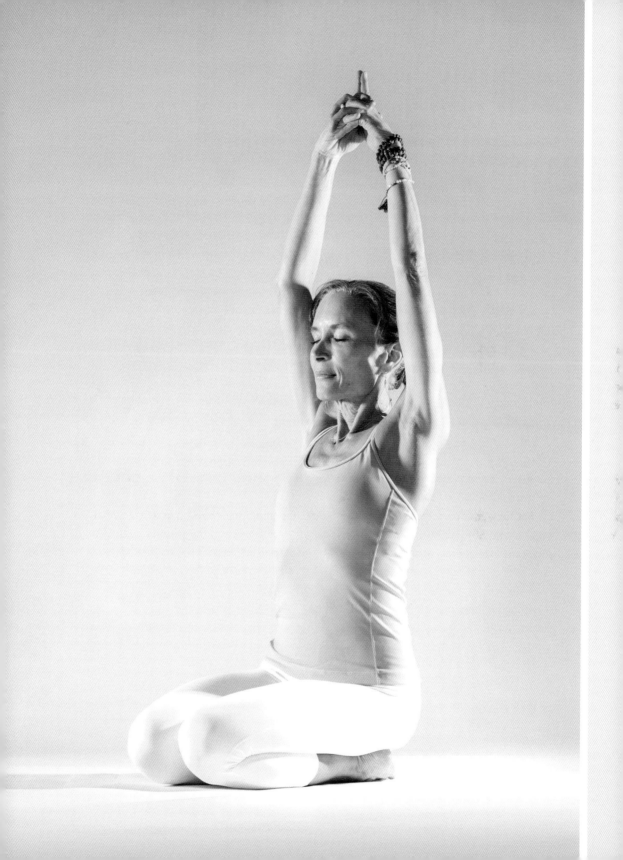

KIRTAN KRIYA

Find a comfortable seat. Lift and lengthen your spine and draw your chin slightly in for jalandhar bandha (also known variously as chin lock or throat lock). Allow your elbows to be straight yet arms relaxed, with your wrists resting on your knees and your palms softly forward as well as upward. Eyes are closed and gaze is inward, toward the brow point.

The mantra chanted in this meditation is the *panj shabd*, and it details the ever-spinning wheel of creation: SA TA NA MA, meaning infinity, life, death or transformation, birth or rebirth. The mantra is chanted in the three languages of consciousness: out loud, representing our humanity; whispering, representing the beloved and the lover; and silently, representing the divine. You can chant this mantra solo (a cappella) or with a recorded version. (Many beautiful versions of this mantra can be easily found online by searching the term "Kirtan Kriya.") I appreciate both options, although with a recorded version, you won't have to keep up with a timer or clock.

The magic and power of this meditation are in the combination of the mantra with the shifting mudra. It is done like this:

SA—the index finger tip touches the thumb tip

TA—the middle finger tip touches the thumb tip

NA—the third finger tip to the thumb tip

MA—the little finger tip to the thumb tip

Each repetition of the mantra is sung and shaped in this way, with 6 repetitions in total: sing the mantra aloud for 3–5 minutes, then whisper it for 3–5 minutes, then do it silently for 6–10 minutes (representing two sections back-to-back), then whisper again for 3–5 minutes, then sing aloud for 3–5 minutes. Each of the six sections is done for an equal amount of time—all 3 minutes each, or 4 minutes, or 5 (with the silent sections in the middle made up of equal periods back-to-back).

As you do the meditation, visualize the energy of the cosmos entering the crown of the head as you chant SA, and moving in a bend toward the front of the head on TA and NA, then out of the brow point on MA. This pathway is known as the "golden cord," the connection between the pineal and the pituitary glands. This visualization is constantly flowing, throughout the entire meditation.

To end, inhale deeply and suspend the breath for a comfortable amount of time. Then sit in stillness and silence for 1 minute. Then, inhale and stretch your arms and spine up. Exhale and relax.

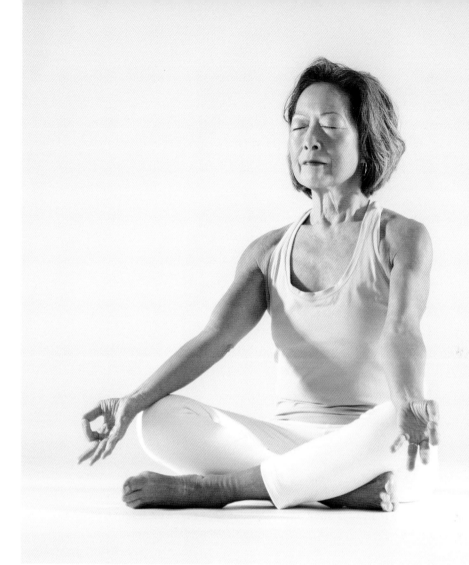

VARIATION TO BALANCE THE MOON CENTERS

Lie down on your stomach with your chin on the floor. Your head should be balanced, relaxed, on your chin (if your neck or chin feel stiff in this posture, relax your head to one side and switch to the other side halfway through). Your arms should be by your sides with palms skyward. As with the traditional **Kirtan Kriya**, you will chant the *panj shabd* and move through the mudras, but entirely silently; the mantra is at no point chanted out loud. Your eyes should be focused at the brow point and again, you will visualize the energy during this meditation as traveling the golden cord. Allow your breath to regulate itself. Practice for 3–31 minutes.

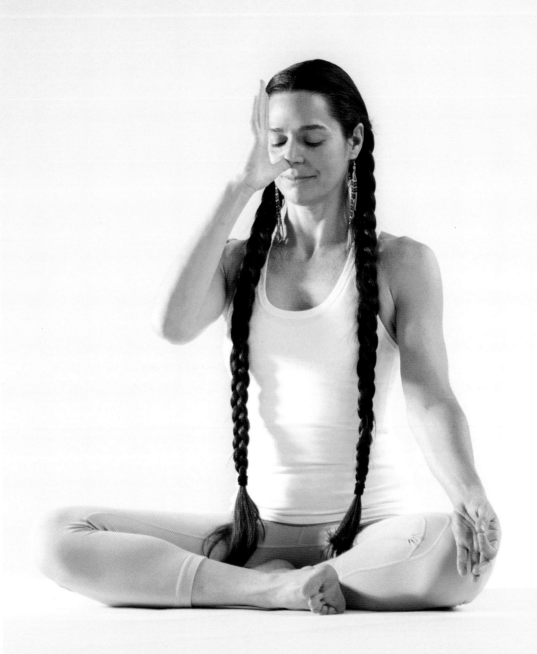

SODHARSHAN CHAKRA KRIYA

Sit in Sukhasana with a straight spine and a light jalandhar bandha (chin lock or throat lock). Take a few deep and complete breaths through both nostrils before embarking on the nadi shodhan variation that is required in this kriya. Use the right thumb to block the right nostril and inhale slowly and deeply through the left nostril, but stop just shy of filling your lungs. Suspend breath here and begin to mentally chant WAHE GURU (pronounced "wah-hey gu-ru") 16 times. With this mantra, you are expressing that "ecstasy beyond words is the destination of the journey from the dark of ignorance to the light of knowing." You will pump your navel 3 times for each repetition of the mantra, in this pattern: WA (pump), HE (pump), GURU (pump). This will be a grand total of 48 pumps, with the 16 repetitions. After the 16 repetitions, block the left nostril and exhale through the right nostril. Your eyes stay open and your gaze is to the tip of the nose. It's very important not to close your eyes.

Continue silently chanting the mantra and pulling the navel as described. To end the meditation, inhale through both nostrils and suspend the breath for 10 seconds, then exhale. Staying seated, stretch your arms up and shake your body for about a minute, moving that incredible energy all around. This meditation can be done in 3–31 minutes.

As mentioned earlier in the chapter, this is both the hardest and simplest of meditations. Begin with just 3 minutes and allow your navel control as well as your lung capacity to build. By not filling your lungs 100 percent with the inhale, you allow some flexibility to pump the navel. It's well worth the effort. Work with where you are, meaning that if you are unable to get 16 repetitions on the held breath and 12 times through is your maximum, have patience with yourself and keep practicing.

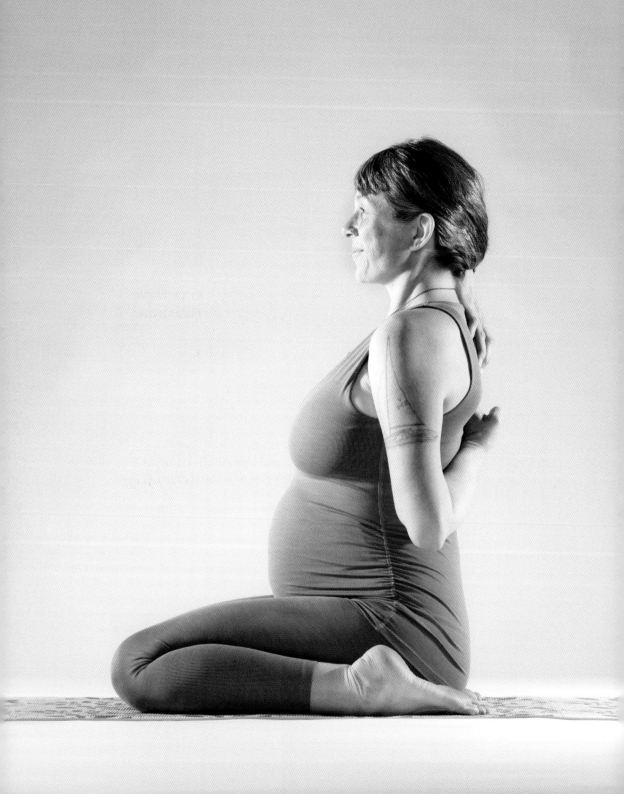

6

We Are All Mothers

THIS IS A BOOK OF YOGA for those who identify as women. Not all of us who identify in this way will become pregnant, deliver a child, and mother in the most traditional sense, nor do all of us wish to manifest motherhood in this way. No matter where you are on the spectrum of intention around pregnancy and motherhood, I hope that you will read this chapter. As I'll explain, "mothering" is about so much more than birthing a child, and the practices and thoughts shared in this chapter can be applied in fulfilling ways to so many other endeavors.

It is a deep belief of mine, as well as a witnessing over the past three decades, that those of us who identify as more moon than sun carry both desire and innate capacity to nurture. This desire to grow something is written into our bodies, coded into our cells—it is both a physical and an ancestral beckoning. No doubt it harkens back to the very beginning of time—certainly, prior to the beginnings of yoga.

The teachings of yoga and especially those that flow from the tantric traditions see the polarity of moon and sun, Shakti and Shiva, feminine and masculine. As emphasized throughout this book, all of us embody both of these polarities. To feel more moon is also to be more "Shakti." *Shakti* is a Sanskrit word that translates to "primal energy or force"—especially the creative force of the universe, the dynamic, active feminine energy of creation. Shakti is both source and cause of creation, carrying the qualities of conception, gestation, labor, and birth. Shakti is also receiving, nourishing, nurturing, and growing, imbued with intuition and compassion.

SHAKTI EMBODIED

Many of us will recognize this aspect of ourselves in our wish to have children, finding deep gratification in this choice—yet, all of us carry the innate ability to mother. The word *mother* itself is somewhat extraordinary, belonging to a class of twenty-five or so words that are considered to be the oldest words in every language. When we trace the word back, *mother* is remarkably similar across the origin points: *moder* in Old English as well as Proto-Germanic and Old Frisian, *mater* in Latin, *matar* in Sanskrit. All of these forms are thought to have come from baby's saying *ma*, which was joined with -*ter*, a suffix that means kin. The Old English definition was "that which has given birth to anything," and yet, one step further, MA is the syllable sound that represents the moon in both tantric and Buddhist teachings.

Technically, "to mother" is simply to birth something, yet deep in the sound history there is also the primal coding of the vital essence of the moon. This is evidence, to me, that we should expand our understanding of what it is to be a mother to include all that we give birth to: creative projects, careers, gardens, art, passions, acts of service, dreams, and more, so much more. Midwifing the unique expression of who we are and making tangible our offerings to the world is every bit as fulfilling as having a child, and for many of us, much more fulfilling.

We can choose to nurture ourselves as well as those around us—be they people, animals, plants, or ideas. It is a prayer of mine that all of us may be sovereign over our choices in how we experience the gratification of the desire to mother. Equally important is that we support all expressions of mothering, that we witness, recognize, and applaud each other on this journey. After all, we are yoked in our connection to the moon. Respecting as well as celebrating the many choices available to us satisfy not only our yearning to nourish but also this yearning in ways that delight and deeply fulfill us. This is one of the ways that we can widen the circle of the moon and walk this path in kindness, compassion, and integrity.

CONNECTING MOON AND MOTHERING

Understanding the phases that the moon moves through each month and the energy associated with each phase allows us to apply our lunar wisdom in many ways. The modern astronomical understanding recognizes eight phases of the moon. But, as we have touched on before, there was a little bit of a slip in the carrying over from our ancestors. In the way that understanding our own cycles allows us to apply a deeper wisdom in multiple areas of our life, understanding the phases of the moon allows us the opportunity to move in a rhythm that works with the moon energy rather than at cross-purposes to it. Consider the ancient agrarian practice of planting and harvesting by the phase of the moon—these observances continue today in many modern farming communities. Whether we are gestating a creative project, birthing a new career, or mothering a child, understanding the way to align with the energy of the moon as she orbits the Earth is rich with reward and deeply satisfying.

As noted in chapter 3, the phases of the moon offer us windows of time that have been defined and refined over thousands of years, by every culture. Almost every single thing we hope to accomplish in our lives can benefit from an understanding of the energy and nature of the transit of the moon. Creating a moon journal to share with your children for tracking the moon's voyage across the sky can seed one of the primary relationships (moon, sun, Earth) within them and is sure to become a cherished landmark in time. In an uncanny synchronicity, my twenty-two-year-old daughter found her moon journals from childhood the other day and it was with deep joy that we flipped through the pages together, looking at her sketches. Her notes on how she was feeling and what she hoped for were incredibly poignant. Connecting to the moon in this way is almost like creating a little time capsule for the future.

Below is a recap of the phases of the moon discussed in chapter 3, this time with suggestions of how to best move, act, pause, and so on during each phase. Honoring these cycles of energy is a way to organically enhance all that we might wish to birth and grow.

NEW MOON. The time of the truly new moon is about twenty-four hours out from the astronomical new moon noted on your calendar. (See chapter 3 for a discussion of the dark moon.) The new moon is the phase of initiation. The moon imbues new projects, new commitments, even new relationships with momentum, vitality, and freshness.

WAXING CRESCENT. The illumination of the waxing crescent is soft, a sliver yet growing. Here is our first growth, a time where the shape and future of whatever we are growing are still stronger in vision than presence. We give strength to what we are nourishing with intention and purpose. Meditation is oriented around our goal.

FIRST QUARTER. Halfway to full illumination, the moon's first quarter is when action is invited. Intention is still held, yet there is active engagement, action embodied. It is a place where obstacles and resistances as well as advantages are faced head-on. The first quarter is a time to apply ourselves in rawness rather than refinement.

WAXING GIBBOUS. The waxing gibbous moon is a phase where the energy is still ascending and almost full. To align ourselves here is to continue to apply ourselves in motion and action, yet also check our navigation and revise where needed. This is the place of refinement and sculpture.

FULL MOON. The moon's light and the energy peak at the full moon, bringing culmination in all ways, both felt and perceived. At this zenith, we have the potential to experience our ability to see most objectively, yet that potential of sight must be chosen or we run the risk of just riding the high. It is at this juncture that we have our wisest discernment of next steps.

WANING GIBBOUS. The top of the moon's descent comes in the waning gibbous phase, as the light ever so faintly begins to diminish, and our action is directed toward harvest or release. Whichever way we step, it is with confidence as well as gratitude. In this light, we understand that even the act of releasing is a harvest of sorts.

LAST QUARTER. Down we go in the last quarter of the moon; recalculating is what is rewarded now. The moon's energy now is similar to the energy of the first quarter, yet in reverse. Rather than raw action moving forward, this is a place of conservation. Movement is accompanied by deliberate consideration of status and success, as well as what we might release and let go of, as we approach the final leg of the journey.

WANING CRESCENT. With the waning crescent the moon returns back to the sliver, the faint. As the light washes away, our actions are a surrendering. Perhaps this surrendering is just efficiency of movement, a release of the superficial and unnecessary, but perhaps we are called to release it all, even the cherished vision. If so, it is done in the appreciation of the value of good compost, knowing that what we release will fertilize the soil.

DARK MOON. Seldom noted as such by the modern world, the dark moon brings a time of thankfulness with which we take our rest. While many might mark this time as the start of the lunar cycle (as noted previously, the precise dark moon is actually astronomically noted as the "new moon"), we recognize it for what it is: the completion of the cycle and a time of integration and reflection. Rest is sacred, rest is holy. To align to the moon on this day is to cease from striving, to simply be. Listen to your body, your spirit—you might indeed find a faint sense of weariness. Weariness is biological wisdom, a soft asking for respite. In pausing here, we make room for the cycle to begin again, fresh.

The opportunity to know the moon more intimately happens throughout these pages, throughout your life. As it felt logical to share the astronomical science of moon phases in chapter 3, it felt resonant to consider the energetic calling card of each phase here, alongside the understanding of the depth and breadth to which we have the power to nourish, to birth. Our power is always amplified when we work to align with the moon's momentum.

Over the course of my life, I have witnessed the deep pain and anguish along with grief and suffering that many women encounter in the journey to biological motherhood, especially for those of us who have felt denied this experience. Much can conspire against us, from infertility to repeated miscarriages to timing, opportunity, and situation. Should you find yourself in a situation of infertility or repeated miscarriage, I would urge a pause of your physical yoga practice until you either carry a pregnancy to term and deliver a child or decide to pursue other avenues to mothering. While I believe that yoga is one of the most extraordinary ways we can live and move in our bodies, as well as being a healthful pursuit in general, there is so much about infertility and miscarriage that remains unknown. To take a break from a physical practice of yoga is to remove one more variable from the equation. This can be a time to deepen your meditation practice as well as to deepen the way you live your yoga outside of a physical practice.

For ease, I am choosing to frame the rest of this chapter and the practices (for the most part) in the more mainstream language of pregnancy, but I encourage you to utilize these practices in ways beyond the traditional interpretations of the prenatal period, meaning that although these practices were curated to support those on the journey to biological pregnancy, I believe with all of my heart that these very same practices could be applied, with intention, to the journey of growing and birthing anything! To illustrate, I'll share an example from my own life. In 2013, I became aware of some fairly dire living circumstances for a number of the youth in the high school my children were attending. I didn't feel that I had much to offer, but I did have skill as a yoga teacher and thought that an introduction to yoga and a weekly opportunity to practice might have value. Fortunately, the administration agreed, and I began volunteering at the high school each week with guidance counselor–selected students. The program was far more successful (according to the participants) than I had dared to even hope. This led me to feel called to find a way to bring yoga to other populations lacking access in western North Carolina. During this period of dreaming and visioning what that might look like, I practiced **Gestating: A Prenatal Sequence** regularly and walked many miles, sometimes meditating, sometimes not, but always journaling the ideas and inspirations that were unfolding. This gestation led to the creation of a nonprofit with the mission of creating resilience through connection and facilitated and supported volunteers in bringing a variety of somatic modalities (yoga, dance, running, strength training, etc.) into area schools, prisons, recovery centers, and more. As the vision unfolded and became real, I shifted into practicing the **Healthy Body Kriya** as well as the **Meditation for a Calm Heart**. At no point during the creation of the nonprofit and programming was I physically pregnant, yet the energy of these practices was an enormous support and deeply aligned to what I was growing and ultimately birthing into the world. I credit these practices with the birth of our organization, Light a Path, as well as leading me to volunteer with the incarcerated, which in turn has resulted in an ever-widening circle of deeply fulfilling relationships.

GUIDELINES FOR PRENATAL PRACTICE

Before getting into the actual practices for the prenatal period, let's review some simple guidelines to follow regarding yoga during pregnancy. First and foremost, listen to your body—regardless of the guidelines that I offer here, you are the best and most informed teacher regarding what is beneficial to practice as well as what you might want to take a pass on.

During the first trimester, our practice does not really need to change unless we wish. I encourage refraining from any pranayama practice that has breath suspension (holding) of any kind or duration. In general, we are embarking upon a time when we are looking to our practice for relaxation and restoration. Now is a good time to begin to become more contemplative and reflective and to step away from pushing or striving.

Western cultural and medical traditions have us view pregnancy in terms of trimesters, but the yogic tradition views pregnancy as happening in two periods—before 120 days and after 120 days. Trimesters are broken into three separate phases, each lasting approximately three months, but a 120-day period is closer to four months. Yogic teachings are that the soul incarnates on day 120 after conception. Prior to day 120, there is a faint and nuanced connection between the embryo and the soul, as well as an influence of the soul upon the mother. Traditionally, prenatal yoga practice shifts on day 120, yet you might feel the call to make shifts sooner. Trust your own wisdom.

After 120 days, we refrain from any postures that have us lying on our belly, including Bow Pose, Locust variations, Cobra, Upward Facing Dog, and so on. We also refrain from any strong postures that stretch or twist the abdomen, including Camel Pose or twists in seated postures. Strong abdominal strengthening and stimulating postures like Stretch Pose and **Sat Kriya** are contraindicated for this time, as is breath of fire. (Prior to 120 days, or in the first trimester, a light breath of fire is acceptable.) Once we've cleared 120 days, we also stop practicing all bandhas, all inversions, and all leg lifts, with the exception of leg lifting when lying on the side.

Lean into your intuition and also follow your body for guidance about what is right for you. Some women find that lifting one leg at a time and keeping their head upon the floor makes Stretch Pose doable for the first trimester—but be willing to not practice certain things right now. If you are in doubt or confused about what aspects of yoga practice are appropriate for you, seek the advice of your physician.

Allow your practice to nourish you and hold you. This is a time when the container of practice can be embellished with lots of rest, attuning to how your body is feeling, what your heart is saying. Chanting and meditating and relaxing are extraordinary parts of yoga always and especially now. My teacher encouraged me to walk each day of my pregnancy, and in fact, walking each day is a guideline in the kundalini tradition. Our bodies were made for walking, and this simple act improves everything from circulation to heart and lung health, brainpower, and memory as well as being proven to fight depression and shift moods. Walking is rhythmic and has the potential to be a beautiful and mindful way to meditate as well as be in nature.

To truly mother something is not only to birth it but also to grow it into its fullest fruition. Mothering is the hardest and most rewarding work that I have done in my life so far. Mothering asks everything of you, including stretching and growing beyond your wildest dreams. Remember: investing in your own self-care, continuing education, physical health, and spiritual needs is also an investment in all that you tend.

PRACTICES TO SUPPORT THE JOURNEY OF MOTHERING

Six practices in support of the mothering journey—whether that journey is physical or manifested in some other way—close this chapter. The journey of mothering is perpetual, continuing beyond the stage of creating and incubating. With the exception of **Meditation for a Calm Heart**, all of the practices that follow are prenatal friendly. Due to the breath suspensions of **Meditation for a Calm Heart**, it is advised that this practice be utilized postpartum only.

Gestating: A Prenatal Sequence is a classic sequence for our bodies as they change with pregnancy. The opening of our chest and heart, together with the strengthening of our arms and posture, all support the changes that will come when we are carrying a child in our arms and nursing. This sequence supports our grounding and alignment while also opening our hips, enhancing our circulation, and building both standing and balancing strength. Kundalini Crow Pose is a brilliant posture in general, as our bodies were designed for squatting, and it is relevant specifically to the prenatal period as this is the perfect posture for birthing.

The guidance for practicing **Walking Meditations** offers thoughts around creating beauty, peace, and rhythm in your walking practice. Walking is one of the most perfect ways to get exercise throughout life and especially during pregnancy. Options for sharing this time with a partner or friend are included as well.

A gentle and effective use of pranayama to relieve stress, tension, and anxiety is described in **Meditation for a Calm Heart**. This simple practice can restore your mental clarity and support feeling calm and experiencing coherence. Due to the active and sustained retention of the breath, use this meditation for other points on the mothering journey and not during pregnancy.

If you are actively pregnant, **Healthy Body Kriya** is a wonderful opportunity to move your entire body and circulate energy and prana, but keep the twisting portion at the beginning minimal and gentle. This kriya is also fun to do with children, partners, friends, and family!

Reclining Hero Pose (Supta Virasana) is a posture that is beneficial throughout life. In discussing this practice I also share some thoughts around the postnatal period and how to resume your practice here.

And finally, **Divine Mother Meditation** balances our emotions and connects us to the divine mother energy within us, the mother energy that permeates the universe. It reflects the central idea of this chapter—that "the mother" is the vessel through which all reach earth and we are all mothers. MA, that first sound that calls the mother, is also a sound syllable that invokes, honors, and represents the qualities of the moon.

GESTATING: A PRENATAL SEQUENCE

1. Start seated on your heels, or, if you are able as well as comfortable, sit between your heels, with sitz bones directly on the floor—this is the Hero Pose, or Virasana. You can create more comfort and add accessibility to either of these poses by sitting up on a bolster, block, or even a folded-up blanket. Take a few breaths here, settling into your seat. Inhale, bringing your left arm straight up, over your head, then exhale, folding down behind your shoulder and catching your right hand or fingers. If your shoulders are tight, you can use a scarf or a yoga strap to bridge the distance between the two hands. Spend 1–2 minutes breathing here. Release and switch, inhaling your right arm up, then exhaling down to find your left hand or fingers behind your back. Spend an equal amount of time breathing long and deep here.

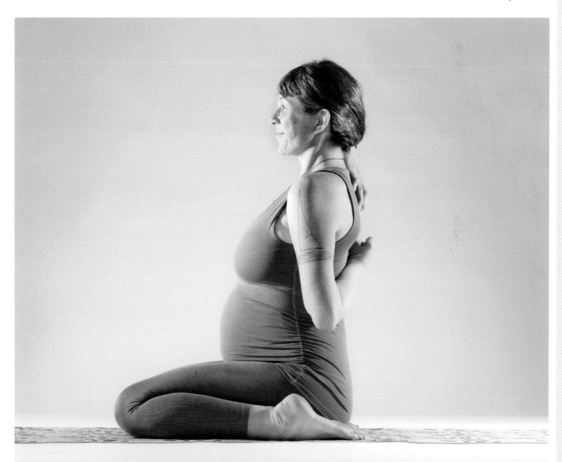

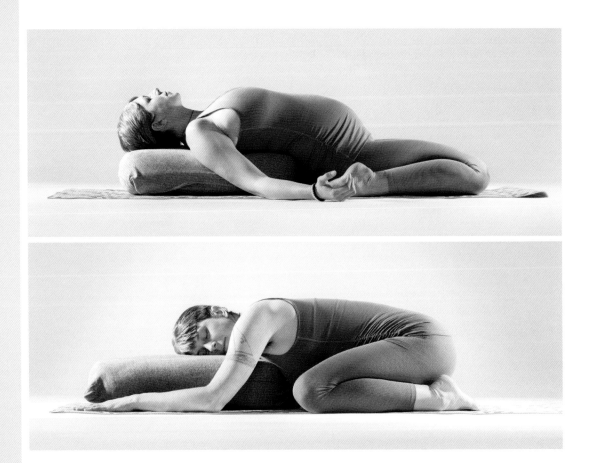

2. Keep the shape of your seat and relax down onto your back. The goal is comfort—so regardless of trimester or reason, use a bolster or even two or three as needed, behind you as support. Relax, allowing your chest and shoulders to open and your hip flexors to gently stretch. Stay here for 3–5 minutes.

3. Rise and shift out of Hero and onto your heels. Bring the bolster forward in front and relax your chest onto the bolster, draping your arms forward around or on the bolster and turning your head to one side. Halfway through, turn your head to the other side. Spend 3–5 minutes total in this posture.

4. Come to a standing position. Step your feet out to hip-width apart, or just inside the hips. Turn your palms forward. Allow reflection and awareness of posture, alignment of knees, hips, shoulders, and head. Ground into your feet and allow yourself to feel the energy of the earth through your feet. Should you be physically pregnant, this posture—Mountain Pose, or Tadasana—can provide a wonderful awareness of your rapidly changing body. If you are not physically pregnant, Mountain Pose still returns benefits of awareness and stability. Spend 2–3 minutes in this posture.

▷

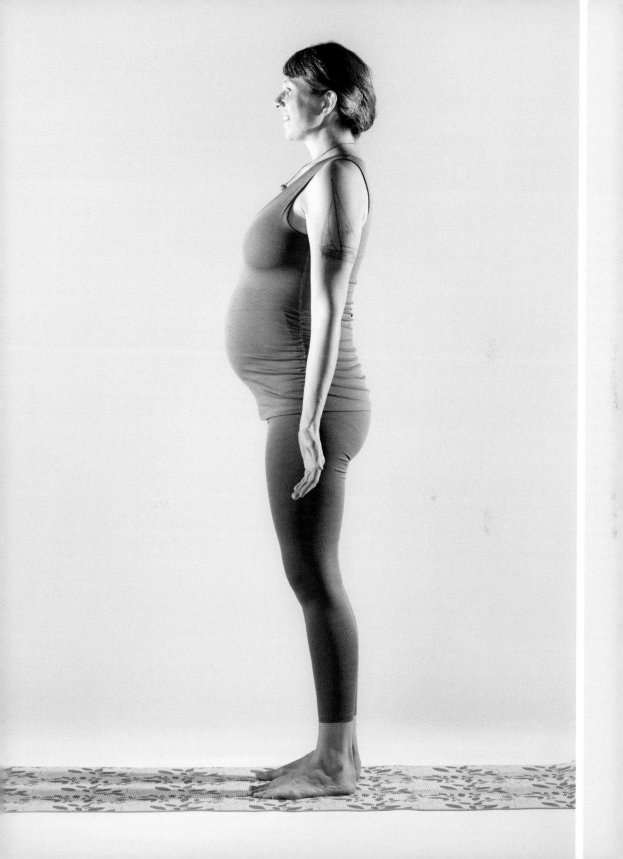

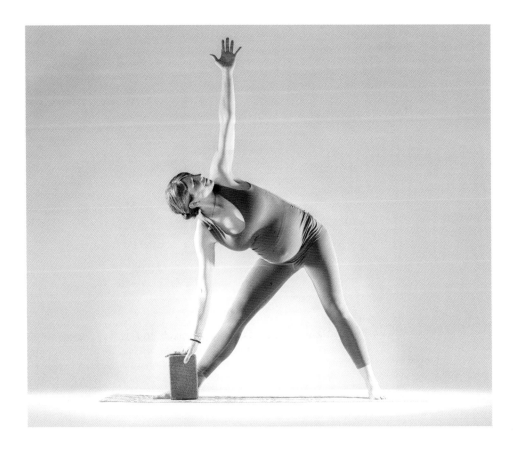

5. If you have a yoga block, pick it up with your right hand. Step your right foot forward about 2½ feet from your left foot. Turn your left foot perpendicular to your right foot. Straighten both legs and lift your arms, parallel to the ground, allowing your torso to open to the left. Slowly fold forward, placing the block outside of your right foot and leaning into it for balance as you stretch your left arm up. If it's comfortable for you, lift your gaze to your left fingertips. This is a modified version of Triangle Pose, also known as Trikonasana. You can also rest your hand on your ankle or shin instead of a block. Breathe long and deep for 2–3 minutes. Rise back up, switch the block into your left hand and take the posture on the other side for an equal duration of time.

6. Release the block to the floor. Standing poses are great for circulation, strength, and balance. You can move through Warrior 1, 2, and 3, as shown in the following photos. If you are in your third trimester, keep your hips square to the ground and rest both hands on a block or chair. If you are doing more than one of these poses, spend 1 minute in each one, also doing the opposite side. Or choose one version and spend 2 minutes in each side.

▷

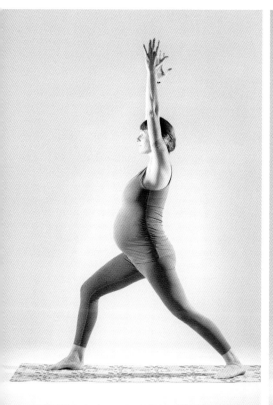

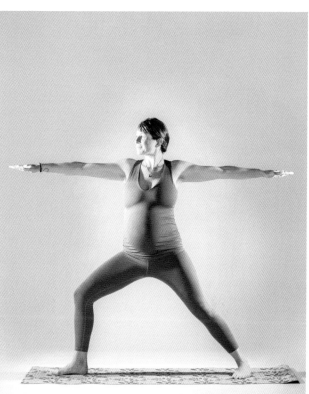

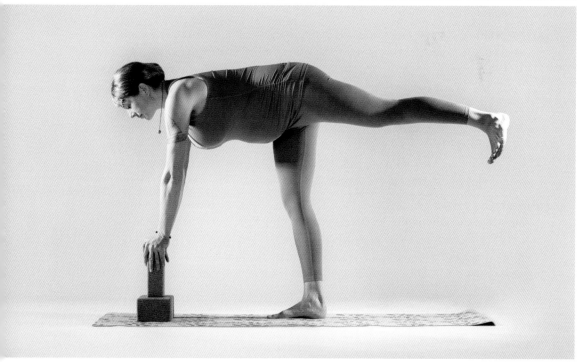

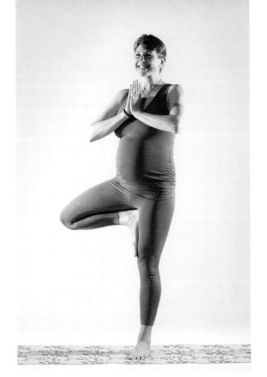

7. Step to Mountain Pose, finding equal balance in both feet, in preparation for Tree Pose, a wonderful and highly accessible posture. Shift your weight into one of your feet and create stability in that leg. Lift the other foot and place it above or below the knee joint, or maybe fold it up into half Lotus. You can bring your palms together at the heart or lift them over your head. It can be helpful, for balance, to fix your gaze on something that isn't moving. Stay here and breathe as long as it feels good. Repeat on the other side.

8. *Important note about the following step in the sequence:* For the most part, twisting and twist poses are not done in the second or third trimester. The exception is this next gentle twist, which does not compress the abdomen or belly but instead opens to spaciousness while still delivering the benefits of a gentle twist to the spine.

9. Begin sitting on your heels, then shift your bottom off your heels to the left, so your feet are now on the right. Bring your right hand to your left knee. Lengthen your spine and turn gently to the left. Don't go far or push—simply open a little to the left. Spend a minute or two here, and then return to your heels and set up and take the posture on the other side.

10. Open your legs comfortably wide. Lengthen your spine and place your hands on the floor in front of you. Lean forward. You can stay on your hands or come to your forearms. If you are pregnant, leave lots of room for your belly. If you're not pregnant, you can lean all the way in to the floor. Spend 2–3 minutes here.

11. Begin in a seated position with the soles of your feet together and bring your heels close to your groin. This pose is often referred to as Butterfly—a lovely image, but possibly imposed by a Western mind. The Sanskrit name for this pose is Baddha Konasana—which does not translate to "Butterfly" but rather "Bound Angle." Set a bolster up, far enough behind you that you can relax back onto the bolster. You are now in Reclining Bound Angle: Supta Baddha Konanasa. Relax here as long as you like.

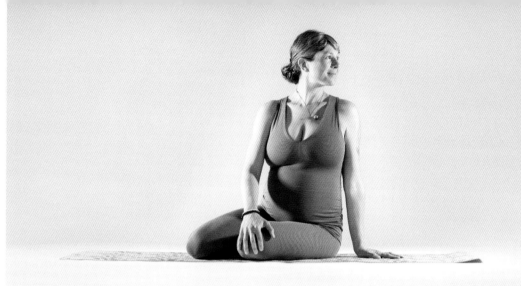

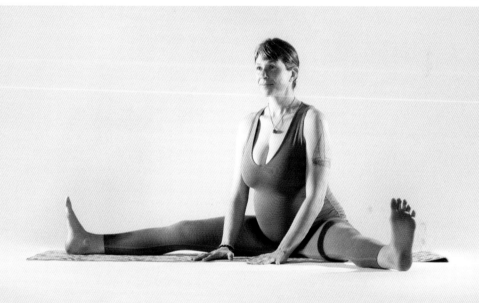

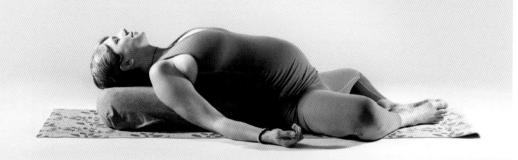

WALKING MEDITATIONS

The kundalini tradition encourages daily walking during pregnancy, and this was something I embraced enthusiastically during both of my pregnancies. It felt so good to get outside and walk! You can do walking meditations solo or with others. If you are walking with a partner or a friend, it is sweet to hold hands and match both stride and breath. If you are walking with a child, it doesn't always work so smoothly to match breath and step but it is sweetened with hand-holding.

You can match a mantra to your steps—any mantra really, but SAT NAM is so easy! I like to inhale, stepping forward with my left foot while thinking SAT and exhale on the right foot step, thinking NAM. In this way, you are embodying and affirming your true self, in an easy and sustainable rhythm.

Many traditions have various walking meditations, including patterns aligning breath or mantra with gait as well as slowly walking in labyrinths. I often found that when walking with my children, for the sake of walking despite having no destination, we would spontaneously make up rhythmic songs that came forward out of whatever we were talking about that day. Those were precious times. The funny thing is that I also remember random events and happenings that were somewhat inconsequential in the big picture but are easily recalled because we made up a silly song that day on our walk.

Walking—even with no embellishments, simply walking and being present with your step, breath, and nature—is an exquisite meditation, all on its own. Don't feel obligated to add anything at all. It's more about getting out there, walking, and enjoying.

One of my favorite teachings on the potential power and beauty of walking comes from Thich Nhat Hanh, who says, "When we walk like [we are rushing], we print anxiety and sorrow on the earth. We have to walk in a way that we only print peace and serenity on the earth . . . Be aware of the contact between your feet and the earth. Walk as if you are kissing the earth with your feet." This teaching seems to encompass not just how to walk but how to live.

MEDITATION FOR A CALM HEART

This meditation is contraindicated during pregnancy and is best explored during other points on the journey of mothering.

Take a comfortable meditative seat and allow yourself to sink in and witness the flow of breath in your body. When you feel settled, place your left hand on your heart, at the center of your chest, with the fingers together and pointing right. Lift the right hand up, palm forward and in Gyan mudra. You can close your eyes or let your eyelids soften to just barely open, gazing forward.

Allow a deep, slow, full inhale through your nose and suspend that breath. Lift your chest and hold as long as comfortably possible. Exhale, releasing the breath in the same, slow, deep, and full fashion. When you are empty of breath, hold that exhale suspended, again as long as comfortably possible.

Allow yourself to be fully present with the flow, sensation, and regulation of the breath. This meditation is short, just 3 minutes. To end, inhale and exhale continuously and strongly 3 times, then relax.

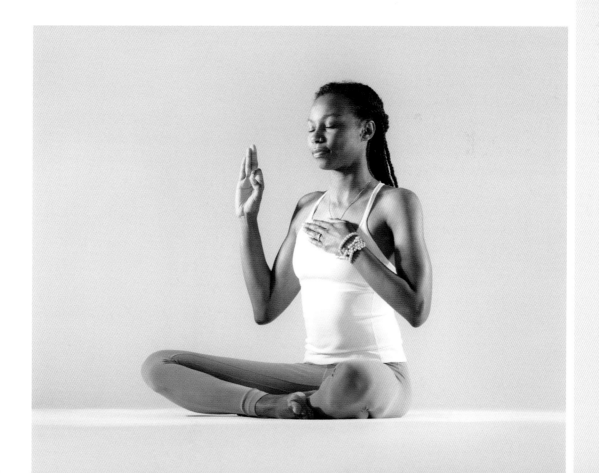

HEALTHY BODY KRIYA

This kriya is a gift from my teacher Guru Rattana Kaur. Allow yourself to either move (shimmy) or ground between the exercises as your body wants. Take ownership of the space around your body, in addition to your physical body.

1. Standing, feet hip-width apart, lift both arms straight out to the sides, just a bit higher than parallel to the ground. Turn your palms so they are forward facing. Inhale and twist your torso, swinging your arms as well, to the left. Exhale and twist to the right. Continue inhaling as you twist to the left and exhaling as you twist to the right for 1–3 minutes. Allow the momentum of the arm swing to carry you.

2. Continue in the posture above but flip your palms downward and slowly bend from the hips to the left, allowing your left arm to come down as your right arm goes up (keeping your arms in a straight line with each other). Rise back up to the center. Bend to the right. Keep going. Maintain an organic, natural breath through the nose. Continue for 1–2 minutes.

3. Step your feet in so just slightly apart and interlace your fingers into a loose Venus mudra, with the palms facing down. Hold the mudra in front of your heart. Bend forward from the hips, bringing the mudra to the floor, without bending your knees. Inhale up and exhale down, repeating 26 times.

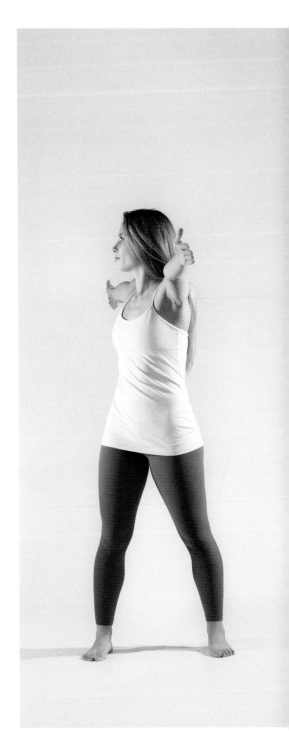

▷

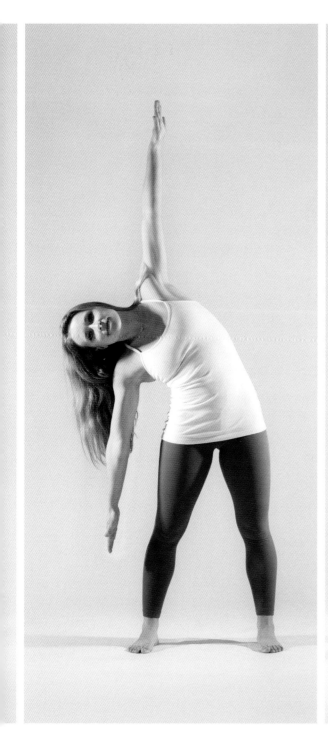
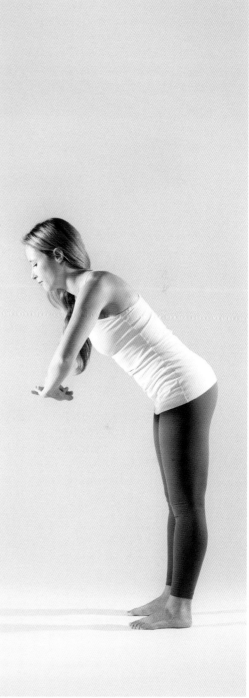

4. Standing with feet about 6 inches apart, place your hands on your hips. Swing your left leg forward and up, as high as you can comfortably go without sacrificing alignment. Return your leg down and repeat with your right leg. Continue alternating, and find the rhythm for 2–3 minutes.

5. Standing, with feet hip-width apart, rise up on your toes, with arms out to sides, a bit higher than parallel to floor. Inhale through your nose and squat down, staying on your toes, doing your best to maintain a straight spine. Exhale through your mouth as you rise up to standing. Continue for 1–2 minutes.

6. Stand with feet together, heels touching, arms out to sides, palms down. Begin to flap your arms in a short, tight, 15-degree arc from the horizon in both directions, keeping your arms straight. Continue for 1–3 minutes. ▷

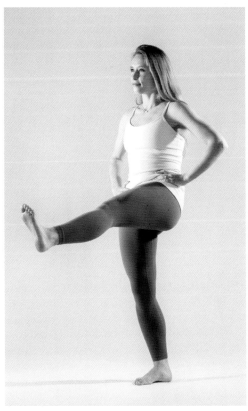

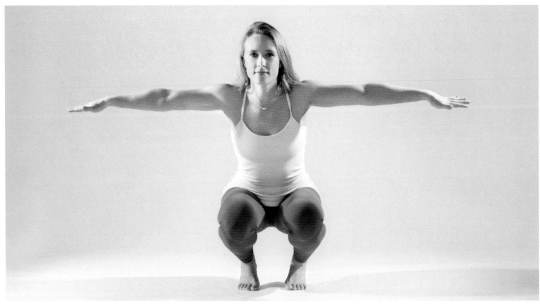

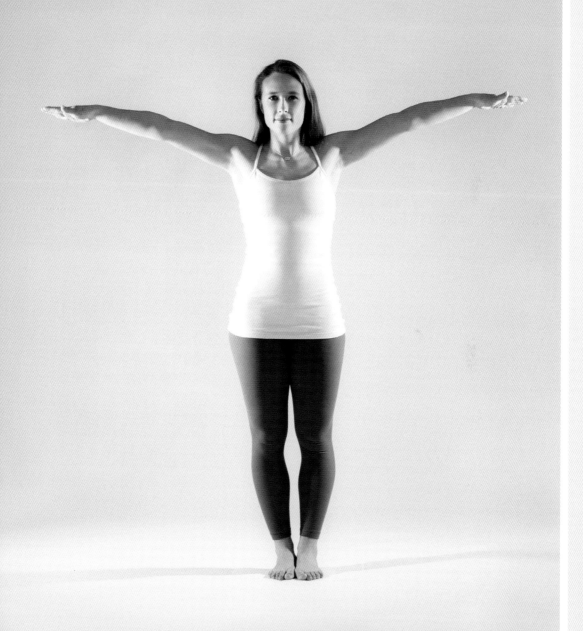

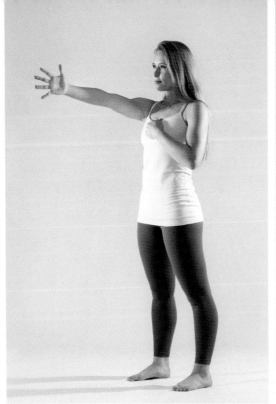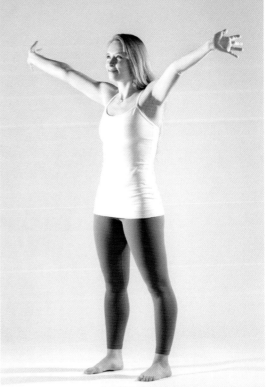

7. Step your feet slightly apart, to begin this movement that feeds the heart and moves lymph! Reach one arm forward with your hand open while the other arm is bent in toward your heart with the hand in a fist. Inhale as you "grasp" energy with the open hand of your outstretched arm. Hold the energy and create a fist around it. Hold the breath as you pull that energy back to your heart—you create your own resistance with your arm, but ultimately you are victorious, exhaling when the outstretched arm and fist full of energy reach the heart. Repeat with the other arm. Alternate arms for 1–2 minutes.

8. Take your most comfortable stance and lift your arms to 60 degrees, palms open and facing forward, fingers spread wide apart. Move your hands back and forth rapidly while keeping your arms stiff. Basically you are snapping your hands at the wrists to create the movement. Find a rhythm and go for 1–3 minutes.

9. Move into a meditation or relax on your back.

RECLINING HERO POSE (SUPTA VIRASANA)

This lovely, lovely posture is truly nourishing to our bodies in many ways, throughout our lives. Virasana, or Hero Pose, which was described above in **Gestating: A Prenatal Sequence** (page 101) is common in numerous traditions. The kundalini tradition refers to this pose as "Celibate Pose." Both Virasana and Supta Virasana, like Lotus Pose, require healthy knees: if you have knee issues of any sort, check with your physician before practicing these postures. You can also create access and support by using a prop to sit on: the edge of a bolster, a rolled-up blanket, or a block. In the seated version of this pose, we create both elongation and alignment for our spine. The torso opens and this posture is often chosen as a seat for pranayama practices. It can also challenge our quads if they are tight and it can open our hips. Mindful, incremental practice is how we make progress.

Supta Virasana invites opening our front body and allows our spine a counter-pose to the often-rounded spine of modern life associated with sitting in front of computers, hunching over phones, lounging on sofas, and so on. This one posture can stretch quad muscles, open hips, counteract the chronic forward curvature of our spines, and support chest opening and shoulder relaxation.

To begin, sit between your heels, with sitz bones directly on the floor, in Virasana Pose. Place a bolster or two behind you, with the short end of the bolster snug to your tailbone. Ease your way back on to the bolsters, let go, and breathe. If achieving

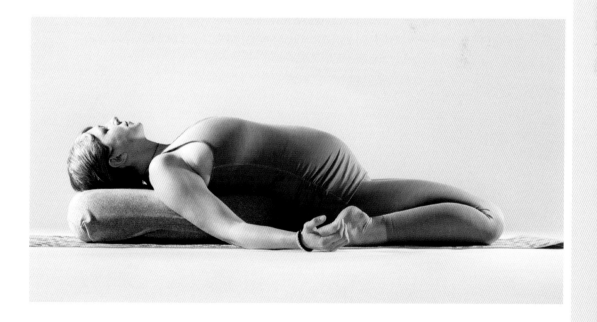

this posture feels like too much sensation for any part of the body, come back up and consider trying again on another day, and by no means continue this posture if you feel any pain. Sensation is one thing, pain is another: practice should never be painful. Pain is the body signaling you to danger, among other things.

Reclining Hero Pose (Supta Virasana) is one of two postures that can support you during the postpartum phase, before you resume your practice; the other is Corpse Pose, or Shavasana (that's right—relaxing on your back!). When you have cleared the postpartum period, I would encourage you to ease back into your practice with gentle and restorative practices and gradually acclimate and incrementally build. Your practice is not going anywhere; rather, it is right there and available for you to resume when the time is right.

It is generally recommended that we take six weeks off (at minimum) after a vaginal birth with no complications and a minimum of eight weeks off after a cesarean birth with no complications. In a world that is constantly pushing us to perform and deliver and work, it can be hard to rest. Yet rest is what this world and all of us desperately need. Rest is how we repair and restore our bodies. Pregnancy and childbirth are grueling, amazing, physical feats. The uterus especially needs to restructure itself after pregnancy and birth, and uterine contractions are the physical signal that this is happening.

Sadly, many postpartum parents are not supported in maternity leave. It's even more important for those of us in this situation to seek rest and repair wherever we can find it. Should you be fortunate enough to have support in this time, utilize this assistance and spend as much time as you can resting with your baby, sleeping, and relaxing. We seldom get a "do over" in life, and perhaps the number-one regret I hear from mothers reflecting on the postpartum period has to do with not resting enough, and instead succumbing to that pressure to get back up and keep going. Perhaps, if you are reading this and it makes you realize that there is someone in your community who needs support during this time, you could offer some childcare, some financial assistance, or some prepared meals or household support. This is how we become a village, how we can "be good family" to each other.

DIVINE MOTHER MEDITATION

For this chapter's final practice, take any comfortable meditative seat. You can also do this meditation in a chair (as long as you keep your spine tall) or even with your back against the wall for support. Bring your hands to your heart, with the left palm resting right on the chest and the right hand covering the left. Experience the beat of your heart, the flow of your breath. Feel the earth energy below you and the sky energy above you. Notice if there is anywhere in your body to relax, while still sitting tall. I often find that I need to consciously relax my shoulders.

When you feel ready, inhale deeply and chant MAAAAAAA for a long exhale. Feel the vibration of this powerful sound in the entire body. Inhale deeply and again, exhale sounding MAAAAA. Find the fullest rhythm for your lungs and body. You can practice this for 3–11 minutes.

End with an inhale, and hold and feel the sound current still singing in your body, mind, and spirit. Exhale and sit quietly for as long as feels right. Allow yourself to feel maternally held, nourished, and supported by the creative and nurturing force that pervades all through time and space and life. You can think of this force as the Divine Mother, or the Great Mother, or simply as Shakti. More important than any nomenclature is allowing yourself access to sensing a flow of unconditional love and support that is infinite and enduring. Let your heart fill with love, and allow this love to expand, filling first body, then beyond.

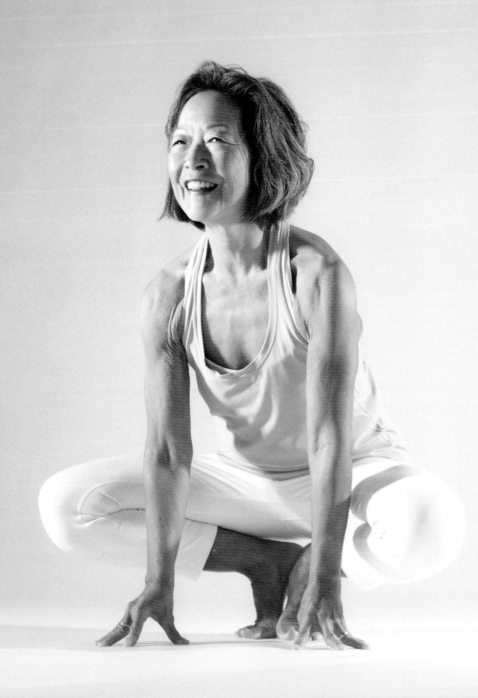

7

Wise Women Practices

RADITIONALLY, the term *wise woman* has referred to a woman both gifted and experienced in the arts of herbal medicine or midwifery or oracle consulting and prophecy. It has also become an expression referring to a woman in her menopausal years—a reference to the veneration accorded those women with many years of practice in the arts mentioned above. While this chapter does seek to be a place that speaks specifically to women who identify as menopausal or postmenopausal, I'd also encourage that we all, regardless of years, or reproductive status, consider the counsel that follows and apply it accordingly. Yoga, and kundalini yoga specifically, is rich with teachings for the postmenstrual years.

All of us are born with an innate and embodied wisdom. Allowing yourself the gift of quiet, seeking stillness and contemplation, is a time-honored means of accessing your wise woman self. Each of us has our own unique way in to this self. For me, stepping away from the busyness and hum of media, news, and what many might think of as "civilization" has always been a way for me to hear the soft thrum of inner wisdom. Spending time in the company of trees and owls, listening to the flow of creek water, or simply resting supine upon the earth and looking up at the sky are among my favorite ways. Dropping into inner knowing sometimes happens while I am flowing on my mat, running on trails, or sitting by the ocean. Other times, in ways I can't explain, under circumstances less than ideal—boom! I know, yet I have no idea how or why I know. Circling back to chapter 3 and, more specifically, the way the moon moves through our bodies in the course of the moon center cycle, I have noted that there is a higher incidence of me desiring communion with my own wisdom when the moon is vaginally located during that cycle. Knowing this about myself, I tend to create more opportunities for myself to be alone in nature during these moon center days. This is an example of just one of the many ways an understanding of this cycle can bring balance as well as power to your life.

No matter your age or circumstance, *you* carry the wisdom of your ancestors, somatically. I can share, with certainty, that the more that you seek that wisdom and create the space for it to come forward, the more you will be rewarded with finding it.

This chapter is for all who seek to hear and strengthen their wisdom as well as for the many, many women on the planet who are on the precipice of or within the years that are considered wise woman years. Around the world, in many traditions and cultures, the onset of perimenopause and the passage into menopause are accorded respect and reverence, and women in this stage of life are seen as being at the apex of what they have to offer their community in terms of wisdom, spiritual insight, and life guidance, all grounded in experience.

DOMINANT CULTURE DOES US NO FAVORS

It is incredibly sad to me that the dominant culture of much of the modern Western world does not regard older women favorably. In fact, this culture often actively diminishes older women and disregards our gifts. The only value we are accorded is through the lens of capitalism—as potential consumers of creams and potions to address our aging bodies and faces, or prospective consumers of diet aids and cosmetic surgery. The underlying toxic message is that our value lies in our youthfulness, our faces and bodies, rather than in our wise hearts and experienced minds. This reduction of women to object is a steady thread over the course of our lives; beginning early, it is cumulative in harm and quite often results in us feeling invisible in our fifties and beyond. The tragedy, to be sure, is not only for us but also for a world that is greatly in need of our wisdom, our lunar counsel, our embodied intuition and compassion.

Concurrent with society's devaluing projections, the experience of perimenopause can be a time of physical and emotional suffering for many women. Our moon times are becoming erratic, our moods are vacillating wildly, our energy is fickle, and our body temperatures are seemingly unpredictable. At no point during this time is it helpful to gaze in the mirror and feel that our value is only skin deep, superficial.

Over the years, there have been various research studies examining attitudes toward menopause among women in non-Westernized cultures around the world. Women in aboriginal populations have tended to welcome menopause and view it as a favorable transition, often with ceremonies heralding the arrival of a stage of life that allowed increased autonomy and community respect. These same populations did not report the symptoms that are commonly associated with perimenopause and menopause in Western culture. Interviews with rural Mayan women revealed that in addition to no significant menopausal symptoms, women in Mayan culture welcome the transition because it also brings a significant and positive status change to their lives. With menopause, Mayan women become leaders and are seen as powerful; their community seeks their wisdom for guidance and counsel. Japan offers another example of the difference in cultural views and lived impact associated with menopause: The term for this time of life in Japan is *konenki,* which means both "renewal years" and "energy." Japanese women are far less likely to report hot flashes, night sweats, mood swings, and irritability—to name just a few of the symptoms women in Western cultures learn to expect.

Could the way Western community and culture view this stage of our lives have an impact on our lived experience? That is certainly food for thought. A variety of other factors can also shape our experience of the onset of menopause, including our diet, fitness, genetics, and socioeconomic status. Of all of these factors, we have the most control over our own attitude and perspective. Many of us also have the ability to take control over our diet and our physical fitness, and even those of us who have less control over these factors can take meaningful steps toward better health.

UNDERSTANDING PERIMENOPAUSE

Understanding what is happening in our bodies during perimenopause can be helpful. When I teach yoga teacher trainings, I often cover aspects of the stages that women pass through and discuss how our yoga practice can best hold us during those stages. I liken what is happening in our bodies as we approach menopause to a skirmish between our pituitary gland and our ovaries. This skirmish is why we sometimes bleed and sometimes don't, why our body temperature can fluctuate, and why our moods soar and plunge. Simply put, our ovaries have been doing their job for many years, and while the age of menopause can vary, the average woman has either exhausted her egg supply or has very few eggs left by the time she enters her fifties. The cells that surround our eggs produce most of our estrogen and progesterone, so at the onset of menopause they take their leave along with the eggs. This results not only in changes in our bleeding cycle but also—because hormones so powerfully impact our bodies and our lives—changes in our sleeping patterns, concentration, libido, mood, and even the shape, texture, and lubrication of our bodies. Meanwhile, our pituitary is working hard to get the ovaries back on track. The pituitary oversees all of our endocrine system, and the ovaries, because they produce hormones, fall under the domain of the pituitary. We all know the ultimate victor in this skirmish! Eventually, the ovaries will take their well-deserved rest and the pituitary acquiesces.

Our yoga practice can be a powerful ally during this transition and well after. As we enter these golden wisdom years, we can benefit from moving into our strongest physical practice yet! Our bodies will respond well to a practice that makes us sweat and moves all our muscles. Incorporating twisting postures into our warm-up and our flowing vinyasa is beneficial; twists are a way of massaging all of our internal organs, especially our liver. As noted in chapter 4, "Practices for Moon Times," the experience of PMS is thought to be a combination of an imbalance of hormones and a sluggish liver. Here, in perimenopause, we again find ourselves in a place of shifting hormones and possibly sluggish liver. Twisting postures stimulate and support our liver as well as our liver meridian. This is also a time when inversions (handstands, headstands, Plow Pose, Shoulderstand, and so forth) can support the functions of our entire neuroendocrine system, especially our pituitary and pineal glands. In addition to promoting bone density, moving into a stronger physical yoga practice can also give us a challenge to focus on and a new way to grow. If we look to the sister science of yoga, Ayurveda, our intuition to step up our practice is confirmed. Ayurveda sees menopause as moving into a more vata stage of life. Our *agni* (fire) is diminished to some degree, in both our digestion and our thyroid, but our practice gifts us with an opportunity to bring in new fire.

Many of us now live in a culture that has drifted from its roots and heritage. If you are living in a community that does not celebrate or acknowledge the new and powerful stage of life that comes with menopause, there are numerous possibilities for you to create your own ritual and acknowledgment of transition to your wise woman years. Incorporating stronger physical effort into your practice is just one way you could create ceremony and ritual, while also supporting your body in a consequential way with both long-term and short-term reward. Should you be one of the first of your peers to reach this threshold, you could create a meaningful way to welcome others when they arrive. In this manner, we can empower ourselves as well as reclaim dignity, peacefulness, and joy.

Yoga always recompenses our effort—in countless ways, be it through better health, enhanced peace of mind, or a sense of accomplishment. I have found, again and again over the years of my life, that every ounce of energy I put into my practice is returned a thousand-fold. My practice is a container that holds me through hardship as well as celebration.

AND WHAT OF THE MOON?

The moon, our companion of so very many years, continues to speak to us as we grow older. As happens in many relationships of duration, the stability and consistency of time we have shared with the moon are embodied as comfort; an intimacy of long-running knowing is felt. If we live in a body that has bled, we can feel a sense of loss as we move away from that moon connection, yet our moon center cycle continues on with us, as does our witnessing, feeling, and moving with the phases of the moon. Being so awake to the moon, to where she is in the sky and to whether she is filling or emptying, has allowed me to also notice when I feel her pull keenly and when she seems to subtly recede away from me. Perhaps it is due to the length of our journey together or perhaps it is my own moon architecture, but I notice how much more drawn I am now to understanding and connecting to the moon's waning, to observing her void. My actions, initiations, and movements are all in accordance with the phases of the moon wherever possible, yet when it comes to more formal recognition, and to ritual, the waning phases are what feel most poignant. In younger years, it was always the new crescent and the full moon, the waxing, that captured more of my attention.

In stepping away from our bleeding cycle, our moon time, loss we experience is more than remunerated by the opportunity to be more present with the moon center cycle as well as the moon phases. I've included two practices for you in this chapter and remind you that no practice is out of reach now. Gone are the years when we might have needed to consider our blood flow or another life growing within us. Instead, we are full of wisdom and can rely on our sense of when to push ourselves and when to seek rest on our mats. **Serabandanda Kriya** is an extraordinary practice, unique in the way that it opens the body and circulation, allowing blood to flow to the entire spine as well as throughout the body. Simply start with as many repetitions as you can and build endurance over time. This kriya is good for the cardiovascular system and our upper body strength. (Incidentally, upper body strength has been recognized as a common denominator in longevity.) The second practice is one that I have come to fondly refer to as **Liver Love** over the years. The title of this kriya says it all. When you support your liver, you support your health in a big way!

SERABANDANDA KRIYA

I hope you love this one! See if you can build up to doing it 26 times.

1. Begin in Downward Facing Dog with your heels on the floor, or as close to the floor as they go. Your hands should be shoulder-width apart, and your hands and feet will not really move throughout this kriya. Take an inhale here.

2. From Triangle, exhale and bend your arms, lowering your chin (only) to the floor.

3. Inhale into Cobra Pose (almost a true Cobra but your toes are curled on the floor and your body is completely lifted off the floor).

4. Exhale back to Triangle on your toes, then lower your heels and inhale.

5. Continue this pattern from Downward Facing Dog to chin to Cobra to Downward Facing Dog, with the goal of doing it 26 times. If you can get to 26 repetitions you can go further, but the practice is to rest for 10 minutes between every set of 26.

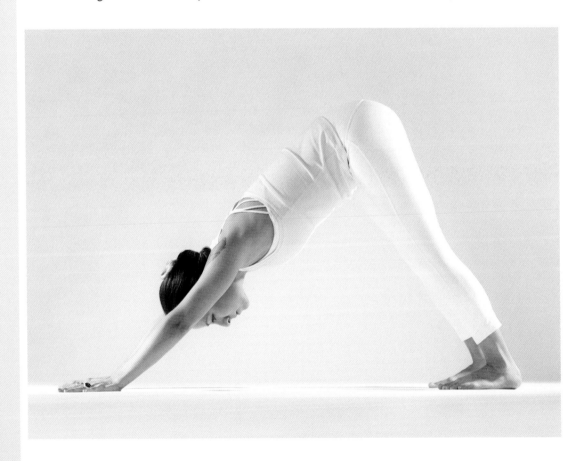

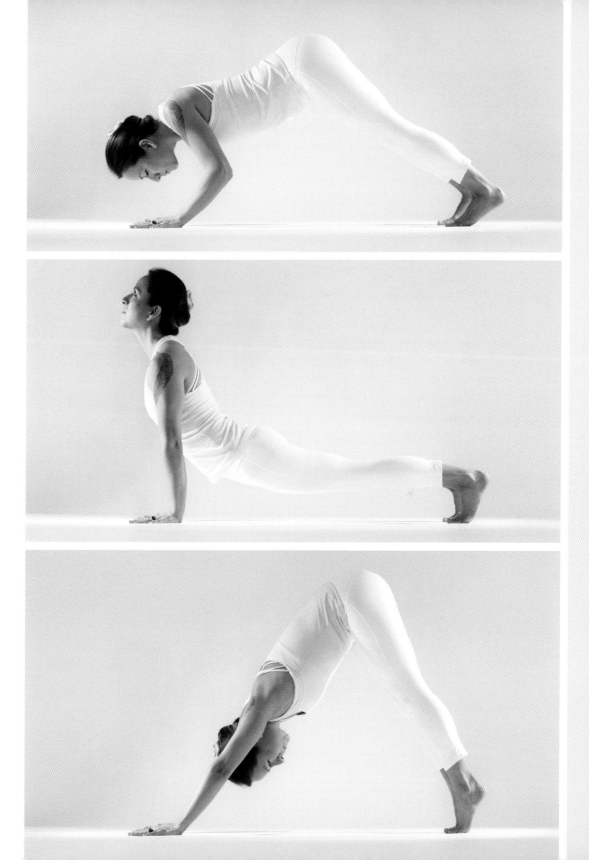

LIVER LOVE!

This kriya has been designed, as the name suggests, to support the liver—and is demanding but deeply rewarding. Feel free to do it anytime! This practice also supports metabolism and enzyme activation.

1. Lie on the left side of your body. Relax your head into your left hand, supported by your elbow. Lift your right leg up as high as it goes with your foot forward, then turn your foot skyward and lift your leg the rest of the way. Hold your toes with your right hand, doing your best to keep both legs straight. Begin a steady breath of fire (page 5) and continue for 4 minutes. (This practice is done on the one side only.)

2. Roll onto your back. Bend your knees, placing your feet hip-width apart, and bring your hands back under your shoulders on the floor with your fingers pointing toward your toes. Gently push into your hands and feet and lift your torso up off the ground. This is Wheel Pose. It doesn't have to be perfect and it might take some practice. Begin to breathe in this pattern: one complete inhale and exhale through the nose, one complete inhale and exhale through the mouth. Continue alternating in this breath pattern. See if you can build up to 4 minutes.

3. Return to the first position, on your left side as described in step 1, and do breath of fire through the mouth for 2 minutes.

▷

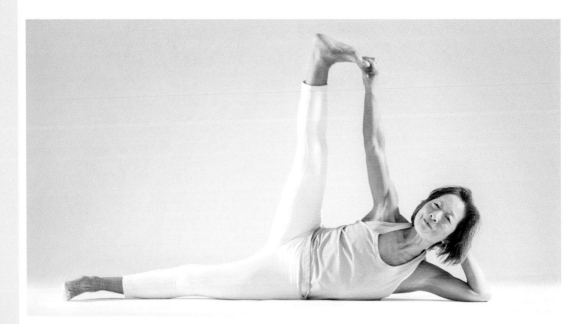

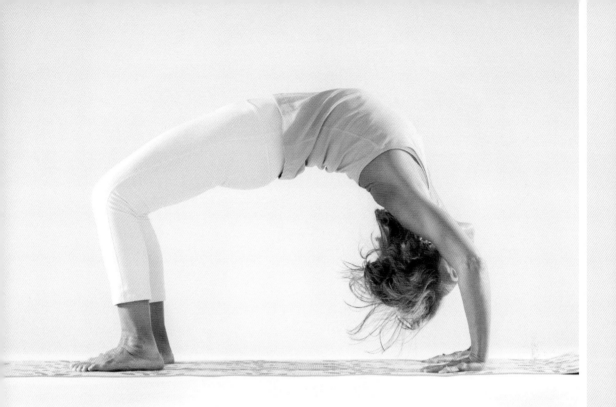

4. Come to a standing position, with feet apart by about 18–24 inches. Fold forward and stretch your hands back through your legs to touch the floor. Relax your head completely. Hold this posture, with normal breathing, for 1 minute. Then roll your tongue into a U shape and hold it just outside of your lips. Do breath of fire through the rolled tongue for 3 minutes. This is a variation on Sitali pranayama.

5. Return again to the first posture, on your left side as described in step 1. This time do cannon breath—a powerful explosive breath through the mouth, with the emphasis on the exhale, as if you were firing something out (like a cannon) for just 30 seconds.

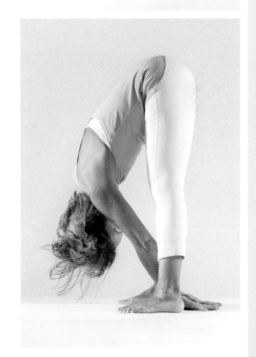

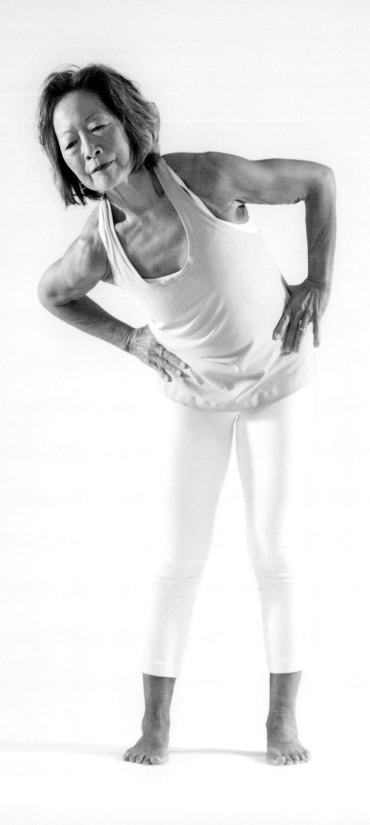

6. Sitting in the cross-legged Sukhasana posture, do your best to stand up without using your hands, then return to the sitting position. Continue rising and sitting, repeating for 52 times (not pictured).

7. Standing, feet hip-width apart, place your hands comfortably on your hips. Roll your upper torso in large circles—just stick with the one direction (it doesn't matter which way) and continue for 2 minutes.

8. Relax on your back.

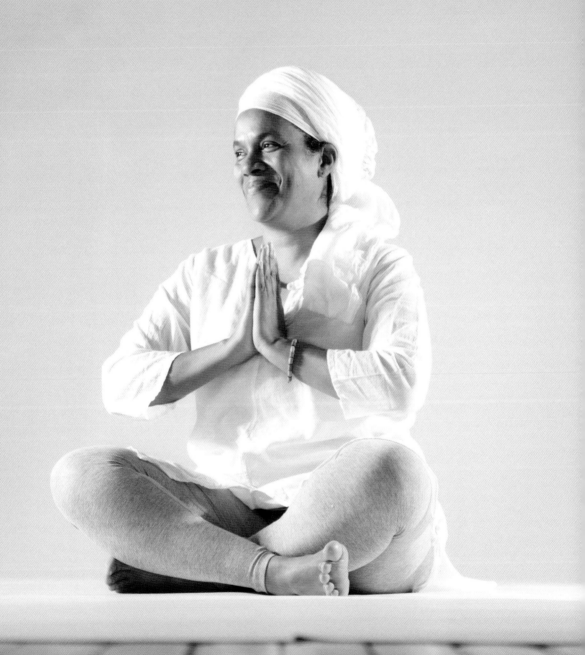

8

Relationships Are Everything

W HAT IS LIFE, ultimately, but relationship? We are sparked into being as a result of relationship—and from that point on, everything is relationship. Shaped, filled, emptied, sculpted, nourished, destroyed—we ride a seemingly endless tide of relationship until we draw our last breath. (That statement is pure speculation on my part; perhaps relationship continues beyond the earthly plane.) The Vedic wisdom that has come down to us through Ayurveda teaches that our relationship to moon, Earth, and sun is primary, the foundation of health and well-being. The Moon Path, illuminated throughout this book in your hands, is a path that emphasizes relationship to the moon, of course. In the chapter that follows, we will explore some of our other important relationships.

IN RELATIONSHIP TO THE SUN

Everything revolves around the heart of our solar system, the sun. The sun is often misunderstood as stationary in this design, yet the sun too has an orbit, traveling around the galaxy, towing our solar system along for the ride. This ride takes about 250 million years to complete, which means the sun has lapped the galaxy about eighteen times since its birth (about 4½ billion years ago). The fact that this orbit is so incredibly long, beyond our ability to really conceptualize as time, means that the deepest experience we have of the sun is that of consistency, of steadiness. More within the scope of both impact and understanding would be the sun's rotation, star-like, with different latitudes rotating at different speeds, approximately twenty-four days at the equator and thirty-five or so days at the poles. The sun also has an eleven-year cycle of magnetic field reversal, where the north pole flips to the south pole and the vice versa. This last cycle might be the most impactful on our bodies and minds. Research studies on changes in geomagnetic and solar activity show that this reversal has an impact on our nervous system, basically showing up as a biological stressor, with effects such as increased heart rate. People report the effects differently, however, depending upon their health, sensitivity, and resilience—all the more reason to keep up with yoga, meditation, and healthy patterns of nourishment.

IN RELATIONSHIP TO EARTH

Of the planetary and celestial cycles that we witness and experience, Earth cycles are, of course, the ones most well-known to us. Days, months, seasons, and years—in spite of our familiarity with these cycles, aligning ourselves correctly in relationship to them is rare. Industrialization, electrification, and global trade all conspire to allow this disconnection. Our health as well as the health of our planet can thrive only if we honor the cycles of Earth. Unlike our relationship to sun and moon, with Earth we have the opportunity to be reciprocal, to give back and to care for our planet.

IN RELATIONSHIP TO OURSELVES

Vedic wisdom also flows to us through the teachings of yoga. The heart of yogic teachings is our relationship to our own soul. Parallel to the Ayurvedic emphasis on relationship with moon, sun, and Earth, in yoga the relationship with the soul is primary and lifelong. To know your own soul is the deepest principle of yoga, a core orientation that will hold and sustain you through all that can and might happen in life.

For some readers, the title of this chapter—"Relationships Are Everything"—might elicit a physical sensation, an embodied fragment of a specific relationship or, more generally, numerous relationships. Relationships with family, friends, colleagues, and—in ever-widening circles—community, country, the world, are as important to our health and well-being as the relationships emphasized by Ayurveda and yoga. We certainly feel them much more keenly, are shaped by them in much more immediate ways. Relationship offers us so very much in this lifetime, with each relationship representing a unique gift.

Often, as a result of indoctrination and culture, when we hear the word *relationship* we immediately envision "romantic" relationships. To think of relationship only in this way, however, is too reductionist. It ultimately diminishes us and narrows our ability to understand the wealth of interdependence in which we live and thrive. Even if it is subconscious, the prioritization of romantic relationships can result in undue pressure on intimate relationships to provide us with much more than is reasonable, resulting in impossible expectations. If we disallow that reduction, we can more fully appreciate the nourishment of relationship we receive from the wider spectrum of presence in our external lives—children, family members, friends, colleagues, and community but also relationships to pets, plants, place, art, music, and culture—which all feed us in different ways.

Just as we are fed by relationship, we are given the opportunity to nourish others. Each relationship asks something different of us, but across the board, showing up with the simple wish and willingness to understand another is profound and deep sustenance. To be truly known is something we all long for.

One of my all-time favorite books in the world is a tiny little book the size of my hand written by Thich Nhat Hanh called *How to Love*. One of his teachings in the book is this: "Understanding someone's suffering is the best gift you can give another person. Understanding is love's other name. If you don't understand, you can't love."* Understanding is fundamental to love—indeed, it is the nature of love. We all have pain; we have all suffered. And for our pain and suffering to be seen and understood, and not judged, is something that every single one of us longs for. You can bring this to each and every relationship. And in doing so, you can witness every relationship bloom.

INTIMATE RELATIONSHIPS

Love is profound, both in the felt experience and in the power with which love shapes us. And as I have noted throughout this chapter, each relationship offers a different container for love to be expressed—so it is important to question default assumptions of romantic relationship when we discuss relationship or love. At the same time, however, it is equally important to recognize that for many people, these relationships are the most influential and significant elements of their life experience.

Pair bonding (referring to a close relationship based on mutual affinity and resulting in courting and sexual activity) in humans is thought to date back to our primate origins, shaping our species over the long-distance run of evolution as well as playing a critical role in determining behavior, hormones, and neurobiology. While humans are not the only species that engage in pair bonding, we do appear to be the only ones carrying the additional freight of wanting "romantic love." Romantic love, in

* Thich Nhat Hanh, *How to Love* (Berkeley, CA: Parallax Press, 2015), 10.

comparison to pair bonding, is a relatively recent phenomenon, arriving on the scene somewhere in the early medieval ages. In spite of relative newness, numerous studies have confirmed that the desire for romantic love is universal for the vast majority of us. And indeed, while our need for connection is innate—a part of our biology that is nourished along a wide spectrum of relationships—the potency of connection that can happen with a partner or spouse is compelling. So compelling that many of us will feel unfulfilled without it, in spite of a life that is otherwise deeply satisfying.

And then, well, sex. The whole sex thing . . . a biological desire that has destroyed empires, and no doubt has upended as many lives as it has soothed.

Let's begin with the understanding that sex can be stratospherically-off-the-charts-beyond-verbal-articulation amazing! Sex can be profound, luscious, generous—an incredibly intimate and vulnerable expression of love. In fact, sex also offers us the potential of a deep and unique communion, a way to merge and touch infinity with your partner. Sex can also simply be a physical act between two consenting adults, gratifying and satisfying as an act of physicality and release.

Kundalini yoga teachings view sex as healthy, powerful, and sacred, adjacent to our spiritual practice. Sex is considered one of the ultimate expressions of creativity, as it could result in the creation of new life. All yogic teachings regard sexual energy as precious, as well as finite. The source that we draw upon for sex is the very same source that we draw upon to fuel our creative output, for instance expressed in outlets such as tactile works of art, the written or spoken word, music, cooking, or craft. In understanding the nature of our construction, the limits of the physical body, and the many ways in which we might fulfill our dharma (a word that is layered with meaning and refers here to our purpose or mission) in this lifetime, we also understand that it is our responsibility to practice discernment, to be wise with how we spend this energy. Indeed, Patanjali tells us, at the outset of the Yoga Sutras, that our sadhana (practice) requires using our sexual energy wisely, with the vow of *brahmacarya*. Brahmacarya is the vow to be in integrity, to be in right relationship with others as well as with our own desires and appetites. With brahmacarya guiding us, we understand that there is a code of conduct and this is especially true in our most intimate relationships.

The ancient and original codification of yoga explains that restraint around sexual energy allows for more vitality and energy in our yoga practice, creating more fuel for the journey to self-realization. In contemporary times, very few people are dedicating their entire life to yoga, yet this essential teaching around the nature of our construction is still relevant. While we might not be overly concerned with having less energy for our yoga practice as a consequence of having excessive sex, we might bring more discernment to our sexual inclinations when we realize that sexual excess could diminish our inspiration and vitality for other creative endeavors.

Sexual energy and desire might feel like fire, but it is actually much more akin to water, an element that is shaped by where it flows and what it flows through. A lesson that is learned from water is to channel rather than suppress or capture. We shape our desire for sex by consciously guiding the direction of the flow. Our sexual energy is sacred and holy when we bring veneration to the way it flows through our bodies.

Tantric teachings offer the sublime construction of sex beginning seventy-two hours before the act of intercourse. Here, intention is what shapes the flow, manifesting through gaze, touch, body language, and suggestion. Anticipation builds while our bodies, as well as our hearts and our minds, are given ample time to warm and open. This is, in itself, ritual, and in giving ourselves to this ritual, we bring devotion to the altar. With devotion and intention, anything is possible.

The most exquisite sex is a union so complete, so all-encompassing, that it becomes a liminal space, the gateway to the infinite and a way of touching the heart of all hearts, a way of knowing, deeply and somatically, the wisdom of the heart at the center of the universe. Or, at least that's how I experienced it. Ayurvedic teachings on sexual union say that this experience offers more than pleasure—it offers a sacred consciousness. In this way, our hearts are opened to love all beings, as well as ourselves. Vedic scriptures affirm that sex can be the highest and most divine pleasure experienced on the material plane (earth) yet the consequences of misusing sex, of being out of integrity, can result in an attachment that strongly binds us, preventing the elevation of our consciousness.

I think that for many of us, certain elements need to be present for sexual union to achieve the mystical and the sacred. Our experience of sex has so much to do with our connection to our partner, our trust in them and how safe we feel. To be seen, accepted, and desired by our partner is a powerful aphrodisiac as well. Sex is rooted in the sensual, in our senses; in addition to touch and visual attraction, the fragrance of our partner and the way they speak to us can contribute or detract from the environment of desire. We too have this power, accepting our partners and creating the space for them to be vulnerable and to come forward, welcoming them to be fully present.

It's important also to be able to communicate about what feels good and what doesn't and to hear what our partner expresses as needs and wants. Our moon centers are also considered to be erogenous zones and exploring the physical locations of them together can be delightful. A number of my students have shared that this was also one of the ways that they confirmed which center the moon was in.

The teachings of yoga, as well as Ayurveda, encourage us to abstain from sex when we are tired, fatigued, sick, or angry. Remember that sex is a physical act and pursuing it when we are not feeling well just further depletes us. Ayurveda offers us seasonal counsel around the frequency of sexual activity—as much as we want in the season of winter, every day if it pleases us! Aligning with spring and fall, our frequency drops to every few days, and in summer, in spite of the sensual warmth and heat (or actually, *because* of those features), the frequency is once every week or two. Orgasm is truly climax in these teachings; it is the point of realization.

Choosing to have sexuality and sex be part of your spiritual path is choosing to make this act sacred. Ideally, the sacred is held in each day: choosing kindness, thoughtfulness, and honesty, and holding the trust of another, are all sacred acts, all part of our spiritual path. This way of being in the world is part of the practice.

Not all sex is incredible; not all sex is holy union and tantalizing discovery. I'm not even sure that it should be. There is plenty of sex that is simply physically satisfying, and that builds health as well. There is also plenty of terrible sex out there—just a mismatch of partners or the wrong day at the wrong time. And sadly, the world is too full of abusive sex, humiliating sex, empty sex, and nonconsensual sex. We can encounter exploitation or violence as well as confusing signals. With the exception of nonconsensual sex, rape, and violence, we have the ability to choose if a partner is right for us. If you don't feel safe, if you don't trust your partner, there is a reason for that; quite often, our bodies let us know that a pairing with someone is not right for us. If sensations of shame or guilt happen when you have sex with someone, or the end result is that you feel badly in any way, no matter what rationalizations your mind might offer, this partner is not contributing to your health and is most likely detracting from it.

Almost all of us hold some trauma in our bodies. The degree to which this trauma impacts us is highly individual and a function of our resilience. Individuals experience traumatic events in unique ways; what feels overwhelmingly traumatic to one person can pass through another person will no ill impact.

While yoga (especially asana, kriya, and pranayama) can address and ease the somatic holding of trauma in the body as well as build resilience, if you believe that trauma is holding you back from being able to enjoy sex, seek out a professional trauma-informed therapist to work with. And in general, take your time—so often pressure and urgency are imposed on us from the outside. Distinguishing our own feelings from the feelings of those around us is part of the process of healing. I've included some excellent books on trauma in the resources section of this book. And I will close this chapter with several practices that specifically support our capacity for relationship as well as enhance our experience of the many relationships that life offers us.

Energy of Consciousness is a yoga practice that focuses on a pervading theme in all of our relationships: our consciousness. This sequence, which addresses the energy of our consciousness and the magnetic field of energy around the body, is also great for building physical health and enhancing our sense of strength and stability.

Meditation for Protection and Harmony is a sweet little mantra that we can chant when we wish to put the energy of protection around someone we love or simply surround them with harmony. Perhaps we are longing for something so incredible to happen to one of our friends or family members that it feels like we are longing for a miracle. This is a great meditation for those times as well as when we are unsure of what else we might do. There is the added benefit of gaining those things for ourselves as we do this meditation for others. This meditation and mantra come from the Sikh tradition. Guru Ram Das was the fourth in the line of Sikhism's ten founding gurus and has always been associated with miracles, the heart, healing, and protection.

Postures and Practices to Enhance Sexual Energy and Connection is a collection of time-honored ways to deepen our capacity for intimacy, connection, and sex as a spiritual practice, both personally or with a partner. This set of postures is not a kriya or a sequence, but rather it is a listing of practices that are complete on their own.

Meditation for Peacefulness is a meditation to help us in times of trouble. Relationships are ripe with potential misunderstandings, communication issues, hurt feelings, and pain—whether inflicted or received. It's almost impossible not to hit a bump or two in most relationships, and that can really upset our equilibrium if we are doing nothing to repair the relationship. If you find yourself obsessed or haunted by something that transpired in relationship, or your equilibrium has been disrupted, give this meditation a go. It restores inner tranquility and peace. With this recalibration, we are able to access our inner wisdom and address the issues at hand.

Sacral Healing, Sacral Nectar is a practice that is equally appropriate for healing and celebration. The sequence unlocks the sacral bowl, frees the hips and pelvis of unprocessed emotions and emotional pain, and is generally good for the hip joints and the spine. It can also be a nice kriya to do in celebration of the energy of the second chakra, the watery realms of creativity. A number of students over the years have also found relief from sciatica and sciatic nerve pain with this kriya.

Meditation for Couples is so simple that you might page right past, yet it is a treat to do with a loved one. Basically an embellishment of *vipassana*, this meditation invites a closeness and enhances overall health and well-being when practiced

You can choose to do any of the meditations throughout this book with a partner, as well as most meditations in general. Meditating together brings us closer and is sweet to share. When we meditate with another, we are occupying the same moment, the same intention, while also building health and peacefulness in companionship. You can also share any of the sequences in this book with your partner, regardless of whether that person is more lunar or more solar. Yoga is about building health, vitality, self-knowledge, wisdom, connection, and kindness. All of these qualities enhance all our relationships, including our most intimate and sexual relationships.

together with a loving partner. While all slow and deliberate breathing favorably impacts our heart rate variability (HRV), going for the breathing ratio explained in this meditation has the biggest impact on HRV.

Circling back to that second distillation of Vedic wisdom, yoga, so many of us neglect to prioritize, let alone recognize, that we have a relationship to ourselves, to the tending of our own soul. In this relationship, the connection to our divine nature is constant, rather than fleeting. Here we find the coding of our unique destiny, the compass for life. While there is no universal way to be in this relationship, quiet time in nature offers a way in, while also providing measurable benefits (slowing our heartbeat, decreasing cortisol, lowering our blood pressure, and boosting both empathy and altruism). Nature is our true home, and it is here that our soul awakens.

ENERGY OF CONSCIOUSNESS

1. Seated in Sukhasana, feel the connection of your sitz bones to the earth. Lengthen your spine and begin to rotate to your left, creating a circular rotation. Move slowly and mindfully and allow your inhale to be the forward part of your circle and your exhale to be the backward part of your circle. Continue for 26 rounds. Return to the center and repeat in the opposite direction (to the right) for 26 more rounds.

2. Come on to your hands and your knees. Knees are apart and below each hip, hands are under your shoulders, fingers are comfortably spread. As you inhale, allow your pelvis to tilt back and your belly to drop toward the floor while also lifting your head—this is Cow Pose. As you exhale, tuck your pelvis in, arch your spine up, and release your head downward—this is Cat Pose. Together, they are known as Cat/Cow. Continue moving with your breath for 1–3 minutes.

▷

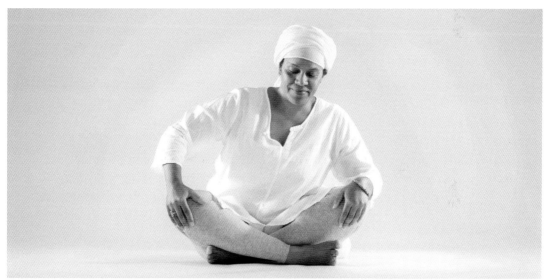

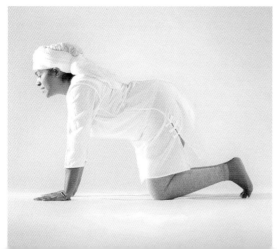
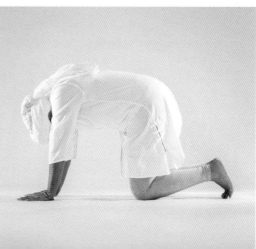

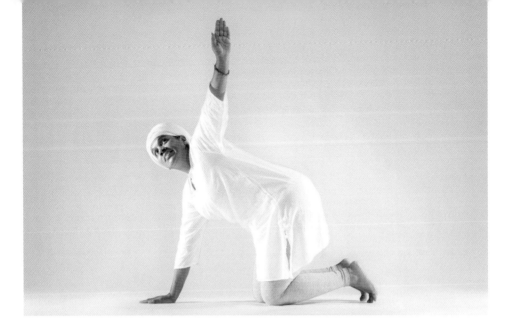

3. Return to hands and knees, positioned like a table. Inhale and sweep your right arm up sideways to the sky; follow with your gaze. Exhale and return your right arm back down. Continue for 1 minute. Switch to the left arm and repeat the process for 1 minute.

4. Return again to being seated in Sukhasana. Curl your fingers so that the finger-tips are touching the top of the palm on both hands. Release your thumb straight up. Raise both arms to approximately 60 degrees and tilt your wrists so that the thumbs point straight up and the palms are forward. Relax your shoulders down your back so the tension of the posture is in the arms, not the shoulders. Hold this posture with a steady breath of fire (page 5) for 3 minutes.

5. Still seated in Sukhasana, lift your arms so the elbows are shoulder level, then bend your arms and spread your fingers wide. Place your hands in front of your eyes, a few inches out from your face. Move your elbows, bringing your hands out from in front of your eyes. Move back and forth rapidly, shielding the eyes and away from the eyes. Keep your eyes open. Do this for 2–3 minutes, letting your breath come naturally through the nose.

6. Return to a standing position. Step your right foot forward and left leg back, with right knee bent and over the right ankle, left heel is down and left foot turned slightly forward. Lift up your arms, bringing the right hand forward and holding it as if you were holding an archery bow. Draw the left arm back, as if you were drawing the bowstring back, taking the aptly named Archer Pose. Now begin to pulse gently in this posture, moving slightly forward over the right knee and then slightly back. Continue this pulsing for 2 minutes. Repeat on the other side, with the left leg forward, for an equal duration.

▷

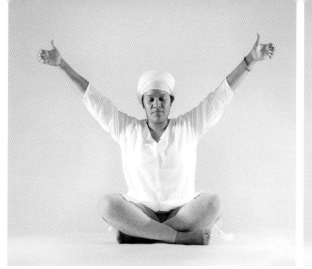
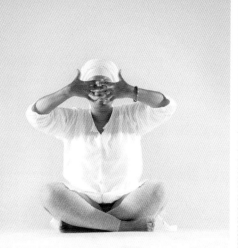
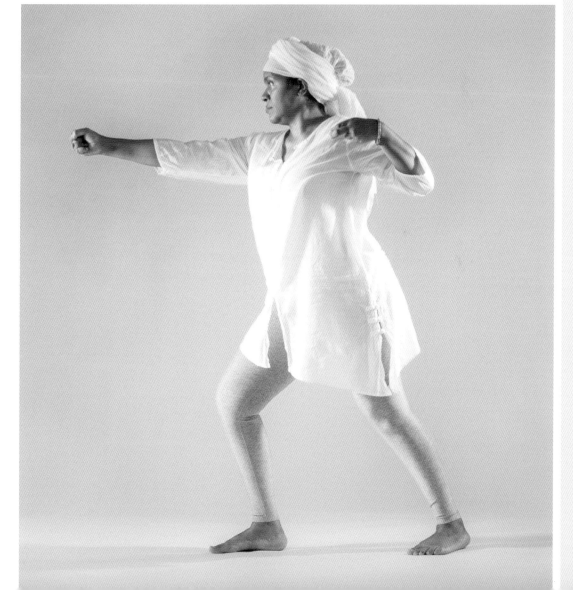

7. Come down on your mat, lying on your stomach. Slide your hands forward underneath your shoulders, resting your chin on the ground. Bring the heels of your feet together. Draw the blades of your shoulders slightly together as well as slightly down the back. Lightly push into your hands and do your best to allow your back muscles to lift you into Cobra Pose. Keep your neck long, heart forward, and gaze lifted.

8. Release your chest to the floor and push up into Downward Facing Dog, stepping your feet hip-width apart and relaxing your head.

9. Move between Cobra and Downward Facing Dog, back and forth, alternating for 5 minutes. Allow your breath to be relaxed and through your nose.

10. Return again to being seated in Sukhasana and meditate, on the flow of the breath and the sensations of the body. You can also meditate on the mantra WAHE GURU: "the bliss of being led from the darkness of ignorance to the light of knowing."

11. Relax.

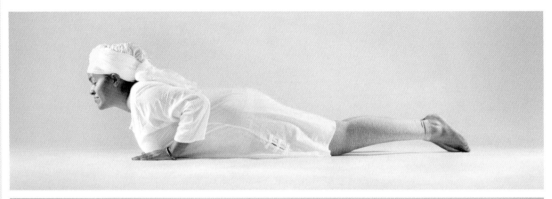

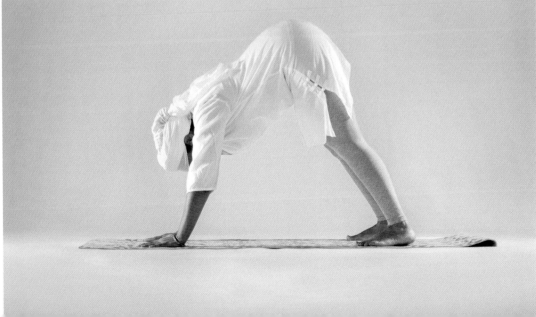

MEDITATION FOR PROTECTION AND HARMONY

This meditation brings a sense of peacefulness as well as a sense of aligning to the greater play of energy in the universe.

Take a sitting position, in any comfortable meditative posture. Soften your eyelids and allow your eyes to almost close. Your left hand will take Surya mudra, with the thumb tip touching the ring finger, and your right hand will take Shuni mudra, with the tip of the middle finger touching the thumb tip. Rest the wrists of both hands on your knees, keeping the mudras but relaxing your arms.

1. Inhale and chant softly, in a monotone, the mantra GURU GURU WAHE GURU, GURU RAM DAS GURU as you exhale.

2. Continue this mantra for anywhere from 11 to 31 minutes.

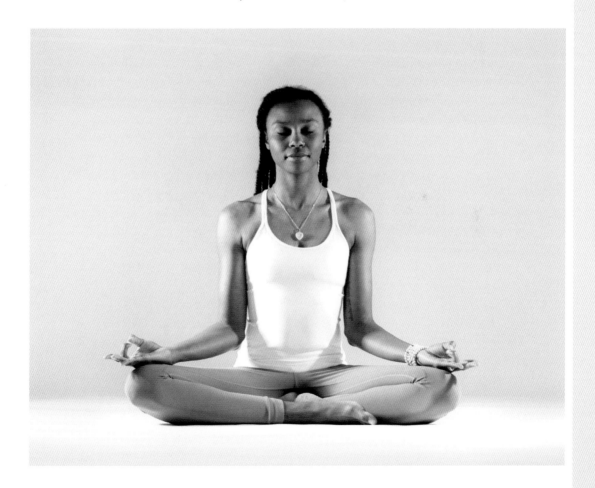

POSTURES AND PRACTICES TO ENHANCE
SEXUAL ENERGY AND CONNECTION

This is not a kriya or a sequence; it is a list that consists of some postures and practices that can bring some juice and vitality to your sexual life. You can practice these on your own or with your partner.

SAT KRIYA! This practice is detailed on page 86. **Sat Kriya**, as mentioned earlier, is one of the most powerful of all the kriyas and is said to address our entire selves, both physical as well as subtle (that is, involving chakras, light bodies, meridians). Additionally, this kriya is brilliant for tapping into our sexual energy and potency. Often, practitioners will allow the kriya to transform sexual energy, lifting it higher in the body for creative expression, yet we also have the opportunity to practice this one with our partner, aligning our rhythm and holding the intention of allowing the energy of the kriya to be directed into our sexual relationship.

FROG POSE! This posture is 100 percent about our second chakra—*svadhisthana*. *Svadhisthana* is the Sanskrit term for the second chakra, which is located in the lower abdomen and houses our sexual organs. This chakra is ruled by the element of water and so has the energy of flow. This is the seat of our creativity as well as our enjoyment and pleasure in sensual delights. When we look at the Sanskrit roots within the word *svadhisthana*, we understand that this word translates to, roughly, "sweetness in one's own seat." To do Frog, crouch down on the balls of your feet with your heels lifted and touching. Your fingertips should be spread and touching the floor. From this low crouch, inhale and straighten your legs, keeping your fingertips on the floor and relaxing your head. Exhale and release back down to the low crouch. Continue, inhaling up and exhaling down for 26 or 40 or 52 or even 108 times! Frog Pose offers beautiful access to full and clear power and energy in this chakra.

ARCHER POSE. This posture is renowned for the way it strengthens our nerves and cleanses our bodies. It is also said to replenish, refresh, and invigorate the sex nerve in those who feel more moon identified and to build sexual potency in those who feel more solar identified. Begin with your right foot forward, knee bent directly over the ankle and left leg straight back, with the left foot at a 45-degree angle to the front foot. Lift your right arm straight out in front, as if you were holding an archer's bow. The imaginary bow is heavy and your arm is tensed. Draw the bow string back with the left hand—again, with tension, as the string is heavy. Allow yourself to work hard in this posture, feeling the tension across the chest. Fix your eyes on the horizon. You

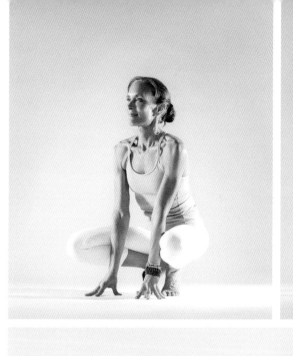
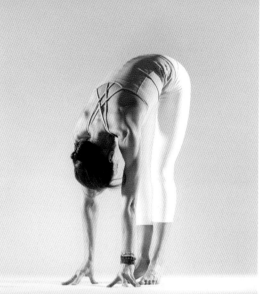
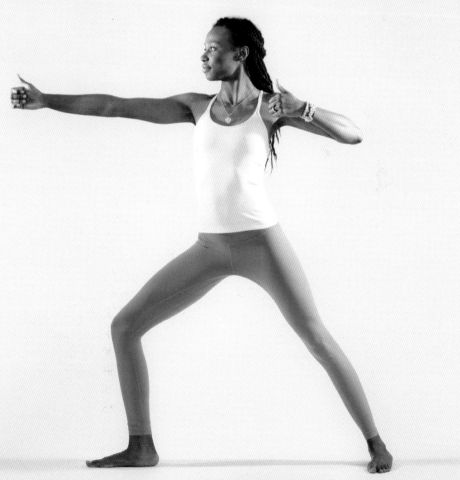

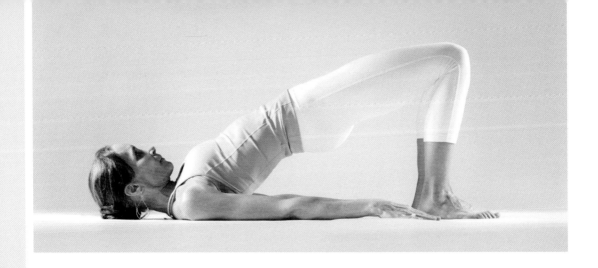

can hold this posture with long deep breathing (page 5) or breath of fire (page 5). Hold for 3–5 minutes and then switch legs.

INVERTED CAMEL POSE. I love this posture and can attest to the ability it offers to access the most beautiful and sensual flow of sexual energy, should you choose this focus. It works equally well for all human bodies. Begin by lying on your back and bend your knees. Knees and feet should stay hip-width apart the entire time. You can hold on to your ankles or relax your hands on the ground. Inhale and lift your pelvis skyward, engaging the gluteus muscles as you lift, keeping your head and shoulders relaxed and down. Exhale and relax back down. I find that 40 repetitions is just right. Feel free to experiment and find the right number for you.

SHUKRA KRIYAS! Also known as **Venus Kriyas!** *Shukra* means "bright and clear," and it is also the term in Hindu astrology for Venus. Venus is widely considered the planetary energy that represents love and beauty. So, right away, from the name alone, we understand that these kriyas are very specifically about love, about being bright and clear, together. These kriyas come to us from the tantric tradition—specifically, white tantric practices. These kriyas are always done with a partner, never alone. While it doesn't have to be a sexual partner, to do these practices with a sexual partner is profound. Shukra Kriyas are incredibly powerful and ancient practices that are meant to unify two into one, creating the foundation for sexual union as spiritual practice. These practices are generally around 3 minutes and we are cautioned to never go longer than the times noted, as a respect for the tradition and the privilege of practicing these sacred kriyas. There are many Shukra Kriyas; I am sharing my two favorites here.

» Sending Prana: Both partners take a posture sitting on their heels, facing each other. The arms extend straight out from the shoulders and the partners touch palms together. Gaze into each other's eyes, blinking as little as possible. Send prana (energy) to each other through the hands as well as the eyes. See your soul in your partner's eyes. Continue doing this for 2 minutes. Then close your eyes, still touching palms, and visualize your partner for 1 more minute. As you visualize them, allow yourself to feel all that you love about them, all that moves you and enchants you about them. After the minute is up, inhale deeply, exhale, and relax.

» Heart Lotus: Partners can sit in Sukhasana, or Lotus Pose, facing each other, knees touching. Look into your partner's eyes. Both of you will form your hands into Lotus mudra, with the base of the wrists touching and the fingers spread and cupped like a lotus. One of the partners will put their little fingers under the other partner's little fingers. If one of you is more solar identified, have that partner be the one who puts their little fingers under the other's. This linking forms a heart lotus. Now, look deeply, deeply, into the very heart, the soul, of your partner for 1½ minutes. Try to simply witness and feel in this gazing, without putting words or thoughts on it. Then, each partner places their left hand on their own heart and rests the right hand on top. Close the eyes and meditate on your own heart. Again, allow yourself to go deep, wordlessly, to the center. Continue for 1½ minutes. End by inhaling and exhaling deeply 3 times. Relax together, preferably intertwined.

FOR RADIANCE, VITALITY, AND GRACE AND SACRAL HEALING, SACRAL NECTAR. In addition to **Sat Kriya**, these two other Moon Path yoga practices—**For Radiance, Vitality, and Grace**, in chapter 5 on page 64, and **Sacral Healing, Sacral Nectar**, on page 149—are excellent ways to support your sexual and sensual self.

MEDITATION FOR PEACEFULNESS

This soothing meditation is good for any time but especially helpful for times when our thoughts are worried or repetitive. Being in relationship, any relationship, inevitably results in interactions or situations that feel difficult. This meditation can restore our sense of peacefulness, which in turn allows us to bring peacefulness into our relationships. You can work through this meditation in just a few minutes or spend much longer with it. Give it the time that is needed for you to feel peaceful.

1. Seated in Sukhasana, or relaxing on your back (on your yoga mat or in bed), close your eyes so they are barely open. Fix your gaze on the tip of your nose (also known as the lotus tip of your nose). Repeat the mantra WAHE GURU silently in this way: Feel the sound WA in the right eye; feel the sound he (pronounced "hey") in the left eye. Feel the sound GURU at the brow point. Do this just for a few rounds of the mantra.

2. Bring what is troubling you to mind for a few seconds.

3. Mentally repeat step 1 for a few rounds.

4. If there is a person involved, visualize them and allow yourself to feel the incident or encounter that is the source of unsettled energy for you.

5. Repeat step 1 again.

6. Reverse the situation: imagine that you are the other person and they are you, and experience it from that perspective.

7. Repeat step 1.

8. Forgive yourself. Forgive the other person. Forgive the situation, encounter, experience. Allow the sensation of releasing all involved to move through your body.

9. Repeat step 1.

10. Let go of it all: the incident, the experience, the mantra. Release it and any strings into the vast cosmos.

SACRAL HEALING, SACRAL NECTAR

1. Lie down on your back, lengthening from the hips to the shoulders with your legs comfortably wide. If you have low-back issues or your core muscles do not feel strong, slip your hands underneath your low back for support. Otherwise, you can have your arms relaxed by your side. Lift both legs approximately 2 feet off the floor, holding them wide as well as straight. Inhale as you bring your left heel in to the groin, then exhale as you bring your right heel in and send your left leg back out. Continue in this fashion, doing your best to maintain the leg elevation for 1 minute. After 1 minute, relax your legs down and relax your entire body.

2. Come to a sitting position, with your legs spread comfortably wide. Catch your right toes and foot with both of your hands. If this is not possible, hold on to your ankle or shin. While holding on to your foot, exhale while bringing your head to your knee, then inhale rising up. Do this 20 times. Switch to the left leg and repeat 20 times.

▷

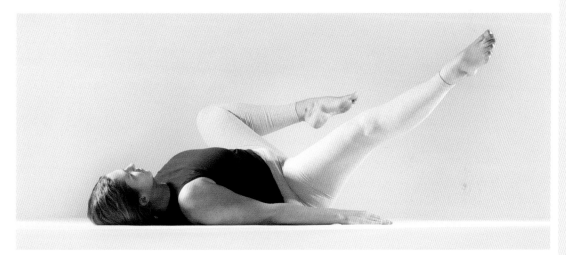

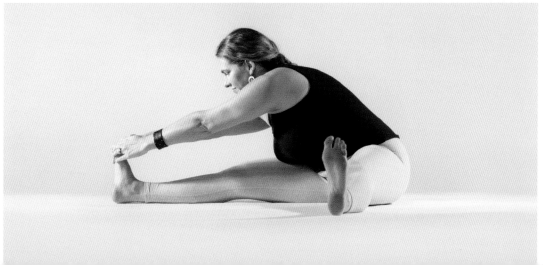

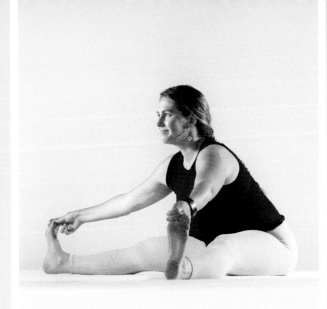
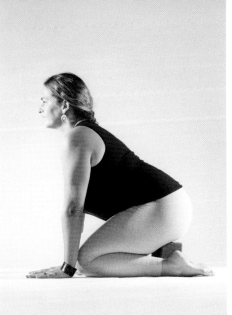

3. In the same posture, wrap the first two fingers of each hand around the corresponding big toe. If it is too uncomfortable or feels impossible to hold your toes, substitute by holding as close as possible to the toes (or ankles or shins). Exhale while bringing your head to your right knee. Inhale and rise back up to the starting position. Exhale and bring your head to your left knee. Continue alternating in this fashion for 20 repetitions on each side.

4. Still sitting with legs wide, holding on to your toes or close. Exhale and bring your head to the floor, then inhale, rising back up to the starting position. This one is done with a breath of fire (page 5), somewhat rapidly. Again 20 times.

5. Shift into sitting on your heels and place your palms on the floor in front of your knees. This will result in a leaning forward, but try to both lean forward and keep your seat on your heels. Flex your spine forward with the inhale and flex backward with the exhale. This is similar to the spinal flex in the **Seated Warm-Up** sequence but with a different seated posture. Continue stretching your spine forward and back, synchronizing your breath for 3 minutes.

6. Relax on your back.

MEDITATION FOR COUPLES

Take a comfortable seat together. You can sit facing each other, perhaps even with your knees touching. You can sit side by side, maybe with your hands resting together. It can sometimes be nice to sit with your backs touching, allowing the physical warmth of each other as well as the movement of breath to be felt physically.

This meditation can be done with the eyes open or eyes closed. If you have never meditated together, it can be more comfortable to begin with eyes closed. This way, you are able to develop comfort with meditating together before adding the deeper intimacy, as well as vulnerability, of holding each other's gaze.

Take a few deep breaths together, allowing yourselves to find ease in your seat, your bodies, and this new way together. Settle into your seat and begin to work toward inhaling for 6 seconds and exhaling for the same. You may need to adjust this breath up a second or two if one or both of you is very tall or down a second or two one or both of you is petite in height. Find your breath signature together.

Once the signature is found, match your breaths, inhaling together and exhaling together. Try to let go of every other focus and thought; simply witness your conjoined breathing.

Allow your heart to soften. Allow yourself to feel gratitude and compassion and love for this person you are meditating with. Allow yourself to feel them feeling that for you. Know that your hearts are communicating to each other throughout the meditation. Our hearts send the strongest and longest waves out from our bodies, more than any other organ.

A period of 11 minutes is an ideal amount of time for this meditation, but you can go for as long as you like. When you conclude your meditation, take a moment to thank each other. This is both the simplest and the most powerful meditation to do with a loved one. Eventually, you can add eye gazing or resting a hand on each other's hearts. This practice can also open up a beautiful and peaceful space for communication.

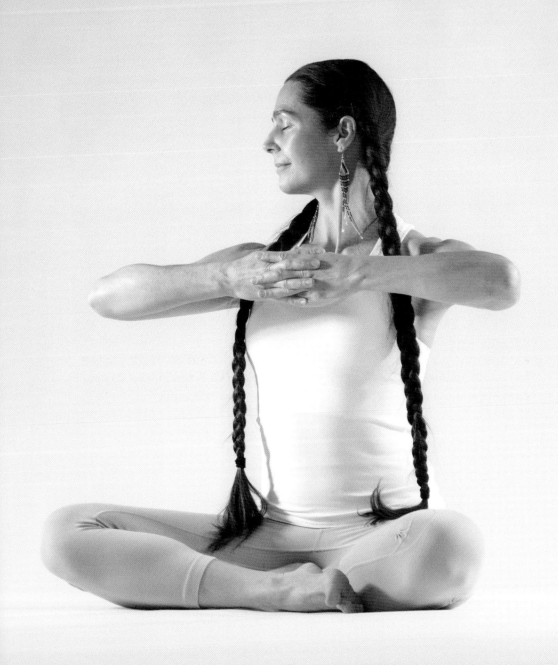

9

Temple of the Moon

RITUALS AND RECIPES

YOUR BODY IS A TEMPLE—for what is a temple but a structure regarded as a dwelling place for that which is worthy of reverence, of devotion? Not only are you worthy of experiencing your own reverence and devotion, to live your life in the fullest, most radiant, and beautiful way, you also require these experiences.

The physical body is our home, our always home and our truest home. This home is incredible, beautiful, a structure of astonishing design, alive with innate wisdom. I wonder if you, the reader, experience moments of sheer wonder and joy, attached to nothing else but being alive in your body? This is what I want for you. If you have these glimmers already, this chapter will help expand and fortify the love you have for you. If this deep appreciation of your body and soul is not already present, this chapter will support the realization of your body as a temple.

The practice of yoga is an extraordinary starting point in temple living. Your practice literally benefits every single aspect of your physical body! Yoga builds strength, flexibility, and bone density; it flushes critical fluids through joints, spine, and organs; and it soothes, relaxes, and promotes the release of stress, tension, and previous trauma that is held somatically. Yoga contributes to heart health, lung health, brain health, and immunity as well as resilience.

In addition to the very real physical body benefits, our practice intersects with and creates magic through our subtle-body anatomy. The anatomy of the subtle body is the perspective on structure held by the traditions of both yoga and Ayurveda, an elaboration of energy and the features that shape energy. As previously touched on within the subtle-body teachings, we find the arrangement of the moon channel and the sun channel in the body. The moon channel is known as *ida*, originating at the left base of the spine and ending at the left nostril. *Pingala* is the sun channel, originating at the right base of the spine and ending at the right nostril. The ida and pingala channels weave their way up the spine, crossing the main channel, the *sushumna*, at each chakra (energy wheel), forming a beautiful spiral, moon and sun energy dancing up our spine. The ida channel holds the energy that is considered "moon-like" for all beings—energy that is cooling, receptive, and restorative as well as mentally and emotionally expansive. The pingala channel holds the energy that is considered "sun-like"—energy that is warming, activating, and clarifying as well as vitalizing for the entire body. Applying the principles of yoga and Ayurveda for our health and nourishment engages ancient wisdom that recognizes the internal moon and sun structures as well as the external relevance of moon, sun, and Earth cycles on our health and well-being.

Ayurveda teaches that ether, air, fire, water, and earth—the five elements—are the composition of all life. The way the five elements manifest in each of us, through the three doshas (vata, pitta, and kapha), creates our unique constitution. The teachings of Ayurveda are a remedy for the disconnection of humanity from nature, from the organic cycles of life. The principles of Ayurveda that I share here are general, applicable to all of us rather than dosha specific.

RITUAL CYCLES FOR WELLNESS

Swasthavritta refers to wellness routines that are based on natural cycles (daily, monthly, seasonally) and is a fundamental Ayurvedic tenet of creating and maintaining wellness and health. *Swastha* means "health" and *vritta* can mean many things but here it means "observance" or "conduct." The monthly cycles are, of course, observances for health based on the moon cycle. In addition to observing the new moon and the full moon, there are four additional days during the moon cycle that we can align to, specifically in terms of nourishment.

On these four days, we can choose to fast or eat very lightly. *Chaturthivritta* is the observance of the fourth day of the moon cycle. It is observed on the fourth day from the new moon and again on the fourth day from the full moon. These days are considered to be times of dwindling prana, diminishing power, and unstable days. We feel the new moon and the full moon, respectively, in strong ways, and the ebbing of that power is disruptive. The most ideal observance of these days would be adjusting your nourishment accordingly and concluding with an evening meditation or simple ritual, followed by gazing up at the moon and then breaking the fast, or light eating.

Ekadashivritta is the eleventh lunar day, in both the waxing and waning phases of the moon. This is a day where the moon energy is extraordinarily beneficial to our health and well-being; the reflected light of the moon is thought to nourish our subtle channels and our heart. Emotions and glandular secretions are in a state of supreme balance on these days. Again, the observance involves fasting or eating lightly. If you are choosing to eat lightly, fruits, vegetables, and milk products are preferred, as *ekadashivritta* observances are days to refrain from grains and beans. The days are concluded again with some small ritual (meditation, chanting, lighting incense—so many possibilities!) and visual observance of the moon in the sky.

There are many ways to connect to the moon and pay homage, both to the moon and your own nature. Following are more moon rituals as well as recipes. I want to again emphasize that this is your relationship with the moon and as such you should feel confident in creating your own ways of ritual and observance. Engaging with the moon in sincerity and in ways that are resonant with your lifestyle, your beliefs, and your heart will always be both the ultimate expression of relationship as well as the most rewarding path of health.

MOON RITUALS

Moon rituals are simply "containers" of expression—ways in which we can both enhance our connection to the moon as well as bow with reverence and gratitude to the moon. Please refer to the moon phases in chapter 3 as well as the elaboration on the energy of the phases given in chapter 6—each of the rituals below can be tailored for the moon phase you are ritualizing.

OFFERINGS. An offering is perhaps the simplest ritual. You can offer your practice (**Moon Salutation**, meditations, chants) or create an altar with flowers, candles, stones—use any and all items of special meaning to you. Sit at the altar and be with the moon. Nature is the greatest altar of all, so being outside, under the moon, simply offering up the heart and mind is one of my favorite offering options.

WATER. Fill a clean glass container with drinking water and leave it outside overnight, where it can be directly in the path of the moon. Drink the water—with gratitude—the next day or add it to your bath.

STONE WASHING. Wash stones or crystals in cool water and then set them outside overnight—or do the same with any items that you wish to cleanse and reenergize with moon energy. If I am doing feathers or books or other objects, I skip the water washing and leave it entirely up to the moon. Most people will tell you that this ritual is only for full moons, but I confess to sometimes doing it on dark moons and new moons, simply because that is the energy that is calling me. Follow your own intuition on this one.

MOON BATHING. This ritual might be my favorite of all and is as simple as implied: simply soaking in the moonlight! I have done this by hiking at night or swimming in the ocean at night, but what has felt most powerful to me are the times when the only thing I am doing is lying in the moonlight, on a blanket, on the earth—just me and the moon.

MOON ART OR JOURNALING. These activities can be done anywhere and everywhere, and they are also the forms of ritual that I have done with the least intention, allowing myself to be "moon led." Try going out in the evening on one of the moon days with a journal or a sketch pad and just allowing whatever comes forward to flow.

TURNING A TROUBLE OR A BURDEN OVER TO THE MOON. Sometimes, our troubles are simply too much to carry, or there seems to be no resolution or way forward. You can offer your burden up to the moon, asking for illumination or simply that she carry it for a while. You can write the nature of the issue down and leave it in the moonlight, then burn it the next day. Or offer an object that represents the trouble—again, disposing of it responsibly the next day.

MOON CIRCLES. Consider gathering with friends and or family, in community, to honor the moon. You can choose from many possibilities: dancing in the moonlight, sitting in a circle and sharing moon stories, creating an altar together, or doing a group meditation are just a few.

ECLIPSES. Yogic teachings consider eclipses to be a time of instability rather than celebration. We do not seek the moon at this time—rather, we consciously seek proximity to a body of water—an ocean, a lake, a stream—or if that is not feasible, taking a bath and drinking lots of water can suffice.

RECIPES

My thoughts on healthy nourishment are influenced by yoga and Ayurveda as well as by the need for lowering the carbon footprint of our diet and eating in a way that is both kind and sustainable. I encourage you to procure as much of your food locally as well as to eat in ways that are seasonally aligned. Choosing to eat lower on the food chain and sourcing as much of your dietary needs from plants is a way to build health for yourself, your family, and the planet. As much as these things are beneficial, I also wish to recognize that this is not possible for everyone for many reasons. If you find that you are unable to do any of these things for any reason, accept the reality of the situation, and do not burden yourself with judgment or guilt. To feel guilt or to judge yourself for things beyond your control will not build health nor happiness in any realm.

MASALA CHAI

Masala is a combination of spices and *chai* simply means tea. Masala chai is a spiced, warm tea that usually has milk in it. There are innumerable recipes for chai, and this is a version of the recipe that my teacher shared. The ingredients work together to aid the digestion, purify the blood, and boost the immune system. You can choose to add black tea and get a little bump of caffeine energy, or substitute green tea, or skip the black or green tea entirely. I've never made just a single cup—I always make a gallon at a time, drinking some warm at the time of preparation and refrigerating the rest. The lovely smell will draw everyone into the kitchen, and you may not have anything to refrigerate after all. You can easily half or quarter the entire ingredient list if you would like to make less.

- 1 gallon of water
- 30 whole cloves
- 40 black peppercorns
- 40 crushed green cardamom pods
- 6–7 sticks cinnamon
- 16 thick slices of raw gingerroot
- 1–2 teaspoons of black or green tea (if using)
- Maple syrup or honey to taste

This tea is traditionally quite milky—you can add 4 cups of any milk you like (including almond or cashew) or skip the milk entirely.

In a nice big pot with a lid, bring the water to a boil. Once the water is boiling, add the cloves and allow them to boil for 1 minute. Then add the peppercorns, cardamom pods, cinnamon, and gingerroot. Cover and turn the heat down to a gentle boil for about 30 minutes. Turn the heat off and add the black or green tea if you are using them. At this point, I like to let the whole pot sit on the stove overnight. (The spice flavors really deepen with a day of sitting, but I know lots of people who just move right on to the next step.)

To serve, strain the tea and return it to the stove, add your sweetener and your milk, warm again, and enjoy. This tea is also lovely iced in the summertime.

LASSI

This lassi recipe is one that I learned from a Punjabi friend who assured me that it originated in the Punjabi region. That has been hard to fact-check, so all I can say for sure is that lassi is popular throughout Punjabi and neighboring regions. Originally, it was more of a savory drink with digestive and cooling properties. I find the sweeter versions (mango, rose water, banana) to be the most compelling, so that's what I am sharing. Traditionally, lassi was curd based, and you can find lots of recipes online teaching you that way. Often, now, yogurt is used in place of curds. Lassi has the potential to be super nourishing, with lots of good fat due to the yogurt base. It is a nice boost for both the immune system and the digestive system.

- 1 cup yogurt (lots of options here, from full fat to Greek to almond)
- 1 cup mango, chopped (you can substitute other fruits)
- ½ teaspoon cardamom powder
- 2 teaspoon sweetener of your choice (maple syrup, agave, honey, etc.)
- 7–10 ice cubes (more if using Greek yogurt, less if using a less thick yogurt)

Everything goes into the blender, then blend the mixture to milkshake-like consistency. So good.

This drink is some nectar for sure! It's basically a vehicle for delivering turmeric to your body in a delicious way. I am often asked if you can substitute raw turmeric, to which I say . . . I'm not sure. I know that in the traditional Ayurvedic way of preparation, the cooking of the powder is considered essential for unlocking the benefits of turmeric. The magic comes from curcumin, the active ingredient in turmeric, for which numerous studies verify claims about powerful anti-inflammatory and antioxidant properties. Curcumin demonstrably boosts brain function and memory, lowers the risk of heart disease, and has cancer-fighting properties. I could teach you how to make a single cup of golden milk at a time, but the recipe below offers an even better option. Here you will learn how to make a spiced turmeric paste that you can refrigerate, so you can scoop out a heaping tablespoon of the paste and make yourself a cup of golden milk from that anytime.

- ¼ cup oil (I like the taste of coconut oil best)
- ½ cup turmeric powder
- 1 tablespoon cinnamon powder
- ½ teaspoon nutmeg
- 1 tablespoon grated fresh gingerroot
- ½ teaspoon fine ground black pepper
- 1 cup of water, max (you add a bit at a time, and sometimes the alchemy requires just less than a cup)

Keep in mind that turmeric can and will stain things, so be careful. Melt the oil over low heat and add turmeric and other spices, including the fresh gingerroot. You'll want a wide, flat wooden utensil, if possible—if that's not available, adapt! You want to constantly stir the oil and ingredients, scraping your pan constantly. The mixture will thicken up pretty quickly, so begin adding your water in a steady stream, stirring all the while. You are looking to cook the batch for as long as possible while keeping it consistent and smooth (with the exception of the ginger bits). Ultimately, you will have a gorgeous golden paste. You then put your paste into a glass jar with a fitted lid. This paste will keep in your refrigerator for at least 2 weeks, but there is a good chance you will use it all up before that.

To make yourself a cup of golden milk: take a heaping tablespoon of the paste and whisk it in a pan over low heat together with 1 to 1½ cups of your choice of milk (cow, almond, oat, etc.). When the golden milk is nice and hot, add some sweetener—

honey is traditional, but you could use maple syrup or stevia or whatever else you prefer. You can drink golden milk any time of the day but it makes a lovely evening drink. Ayurveda sees this beverage as having *rasayana* qualities—rejuvenating, restoring vitality. Drinking it in the evening allows our bodies to have the entire night to absorb the goodness.

CLEANSING BEET CASSEROLE

The earthy, floral flavor of beets and the gorgeous, rich color of them come together delightfully in this dish. This is one of my favorite dishes to prepare, share, and eat! Beets are pretty impressive, packing lots of vitamins and minerals into very few calories. Beets have been shown to reduce inflammation, keep blood pressure low, boost athletic performance, and even keep our brains healthy. Our bodies are set up to cleanse and detoxify regularly; what we need is not so much to consume cleansing or detoxifying drinks or foods, but more to consume plenty of nourishment for the organs that are doing the work of cleansing in the body. Beets are a superstar on this front!

- 1–2 bunches of beets (the more the better), with or without greens
- 1 pound of carrots
- 1 onion chopped, or 1 bunch of green onions, chopped
- 3–4 garlic gloves, diced small
- Olive oil
- Sea salt and fresh ground black pepper to taste
- Optional toppings include nutritional yeast, sliced tomatoes, fresh herbs (like basil and thyme), or grated cheese

Wash your veggies well, scrubbing but not taking off the skins. In preparing the beets, you can rinse and include the beet greens or leave them out. I do both, depending on my mood: beet greens are sort of a superfood in their own right, so I include them when I am feeling especially virtuous but I leave them out when I simply crave the clarity of the beet taste. Fill a pot with water and gently boil the beets whole for about 20 minutes (if using the greens, put them in at the same time, chopped small). Add the whole carrots, or if they are very large, halve them. Now, keep an eye on things. You want the carrots to be tender but also still crisp—usually another 15 minutes but sometimes just 10 minutes. Next drain the water (or save it for soup stock) and remove the skins of the beets. Grate both the beets and the carrots, going for the coarsest option. Toss the grated veggies together in a bowl. Sauté the onions and garlic in the olive oil, then stir the sautéed mixture into the shredded mixture. Put everything into a casserole dish and choose one of the toppings listed or improvise your own. Place in a high oven or under a broiler until everything is nice and hot. Voila! An incredibly nutrient-dense meal to enjoy.

KITCHARI

This dish originates from South Asia and is a foundation of Ayurvedic cooking: Kitchari is a basic recipe that can be embellished endlessly, and you only need one big pot to prepare it. The heart of this dish is the combination of basmati rice and mung beans, which together create a balanced protein that is easy to digest and is considered tridoshic (nourishing all three doshas), creating balance of all five elements within your constitution. This is a good dish for rebuilding your vitality and core energy and also a good option for a monodiet, should you wish to give your system a break.

- 2 tablespoons oil (olive oil works but coconut oil can be nice too)
- 2 teaspoons cumin seeds
- 2 teaspoons fenugreek seeds
- 2 teaspoons turmeric
- 1 teaspoon cumin
- 1 teaspoon coriander
- ¼ cup grated fresh gingerroot
- Ground pepper and sea salt to taste
- 2 medium onions, chopped
- 2 cups mung beans (whole green mung beans are preferable but split yellow mung beans work well too)
- 1 cup basmati rice (or brown rice)
- 3–5 cups of chopped veggies
- 8 cups of water or clear soup stock

In a large pot, heat the oil and add all of the ingredients up to the onions. Stir until the ingredients are golden and the air is fragrant. Add the onions and stir until onions are tender. Add mung beans, rice, and veggies. Stir well, until all the vegetables are coated in oil and spices. I have a heavy hand with fats and oils, so I often add more oil at this point. Stir again and then add your 8 cups of liquid. Bring to a boil and then cover with a lid, reduce to a simmer, and cook for about 50–60 minutes—until the rice and beans have absorbed almost all of the liquid but the mixture is still a little soupy. Serve up in bowls and enjoy. You can top with yogurt for a contrast in temperature and texture.

If you are new to fixing kitchari, preparing it with blander veggies at first can give you an idea of where you want to embellish and experiment. Zucchini is brilliant, as are cauliflower and carrots. Making kitchari is also an opportunity to clean out your vegetable drawer.

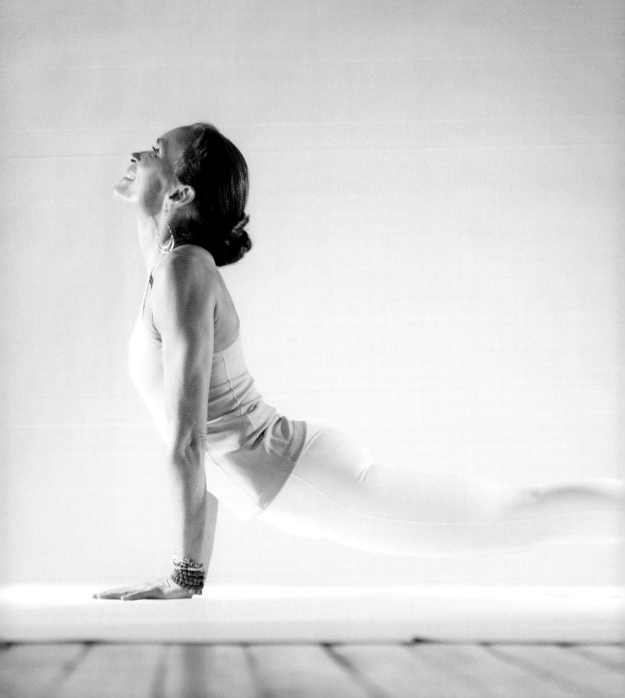

10

Yoga Is a Call to Action

I N EVERY ENDING, there is always the seed of beginning. Like the moon and the path she perpetually arcs, we travel from dark to illuminated, again and again. Along the way, we note the murmur of ancient wisdom that comes forward when we allow ourselves harmony with moon, sun, and Earth, with the natural world. We thrill in the knowing of our bones that the path is less about destination and more about voyage.

Our yoga practice has the potential to heal and restore wholeness not only for ourselves but also for the world. Indeed, this revelation and call to action is at the very heart of the practice, waiting to be discovered and embodied.

The word *yoga* means "to yoke." We practice as a means to yoke our body, mind, and spirit, and we practice to yoke our individual consciousness to the divine and universal consciousness. In this way, we are returned to our true nature, remembering that we are connected, not only to the divine but to each other. Any sense of being separate is an illusion.

Yoga offers us the means to experience unity within ourselves and with the larger world. How we begin has been illuminated for us in the Yoga Sutras. Patanjali, author of the sutras, details the beginning path of yoga, also known as the eight-limbed path. These eight limbs provide a template as well as the ethical foundation of yoga, and they ask us to give ourselves fully to the practice. The eight limbs are *yama, niyama, asana, pranayama, pratayahara, dharana, dhyana,* and *samadhi.* When we choose to practice yoga, we are also taking these vows, and in doing so, the sutras assure that the impurities of our material existence will dwindle away and that clear sight and wisdom will take their place. With practice, we will see clearly.

These eight limbs are meant to be practiced in chorus, and in equal measure. Yet, so often, the Western and commodified presentation of yoga simply involves asana.

Or, marginally better, yoga is presented as a combination of asana, pranayama, and perhaps meditation. And this makes me profoundly sad. It's irresponsible as well as disrespectful to strip yoga of its larger purpose and meaning. Diminishing the practice in this way has allowed the door to swing open to flagrant appropriation of South Asian culture and spiritual practice. In reducing yoga to just exercise, commodification has been both easy and rampant. Yoga in the West is now a multibillion-dollar industry that feeds on promoting thin, wealthy, and hyper-flexible white bodies as the norm. As a practice, yoga holds the keys to right relationship to oneself and the world, but the subjugation of the practice to capitalism (which is embedded with white supremacy) has resulted in a massive misunderstanding of yoga in the West. At the same time, Westernized yoga has allowed an accumulation of wealth in the hands of those who perpetuate this discouraging misrepresentation as well as creating an environment that is elite, inaccessible, and exclusive. This is in direct conflict with the teachings of yoga as well as contrary to the spiritual teachings of the practice.

Yoga is not religious, but as a path of union it touches our spirit in deep ways and has the potential—as well as the stated aim—to awaken us spiritually. In her book *Embrace Yoga's Roots*, Susanna Barkataki reminds us, "Yoga is not under the purview of any one religion, but developed alongside Śramana traditions that emerged as Jain and Buddhist as well as Vedic and Hindu traditions and later was influenced by Islam and Christianity."*

As Susanna points out, the stated aim of yoga is to awaken spiritually. To limit your practice and your understanding to just the physical aspect (asana) of yoga is a great disservice to yourself as well as an appropriation of the practice. For many people, asana is the way in to a yoga practice, but falling in love with the physical movement of asana—with the flow of breath through our bodies, with the sensations of well-being and harmony that can result from asana—is just the beginning. So very much more is asked of us—indeed, required of us—to truly practice yoga in a responsible way, with attention to all eight limbs, to the great and universal vows.

Yama is the first of the eight limbs, and it is through yama that we learn how to conduct ourselves ethically with the world. Yama has five sublimbs: *ahimsa* (nonviolence), *satya* (truth), *asteya* (nonstealing), *brahmacharya* (restraint), and *aparigraha* (nongreed). As part of a conscientious yoga practice, we apply ourselves each and every day to these vows. Each action is informed by these precepts. As part of my

---

* Susanna Barkataki, *Embrace Yoga's Roots: Courageous Ways to Deepen Your Yoga Practice* (Orlando, FL: Ignite Yoga and Wellness Institute, 2020), 13.

practice, I strive to not harm, to be honest, to not take from others, to practice integrity in relationship, and to not take more than I need. It is a practice, not a perfect. With my current understanding as well as my lifestyle, it does not seem that I will master the beginning path in this lifetime. The reality is that, in spite of our best efforts, we can create harm (the act of putting gasoline in our cars is an act of supreme violence against all life), we do not always know the truth, we can unknowingly consume goods that are in some way sourced in exploitation, we can fall from reliability in relationship, and we can take more than we need. The yamas are hard vows but they are good ones, and they offer us navigation in our relationship with the world and each other.

The second limb, niyama, instructs our relationship with ourselves: it consists of *saucha* (cleanliness), *santosha* (contentment), *tapas* (purifying heat), *svadhya* (study), and *isvharapranidan* (relinquishing the fruit of our actions). In practicing niyama, we make a conscious effort to live cleanly in both body and mind, to be content with each day that we are given, to periodically cleanse our bodies, to study the teachings and texts of yoga, and (with the best of our knowledge in any given moment) to take right action and relinquish any attachment to outcome.

Asana and pranayama are perhaps the two most familiar and comfortable limbs for many of us. We take postures and we work with our breath.

Pratayahara reminds us to be aware of our senses and to not allow our senses to pull us from our practice.

Dharana calls for fixing our focus, our concentration, and like all of the limbs, it applies not only to fixing our focus on the mat but also to fixing our focus off the mat, in life.

Dhyana is meditation, perhaps one of the sweetest limbs but also, for many, the most challenging.

And the final limb is samadhi, or divine union, in which we are connected, inside and out, to all life. Samadhi is perhaps best described as that state of flow where we are so absorbed in our practice and the taste of union that everything else falls away.

To be in responsible relationship with the practice of yoga, we embrace these eight limbs and do our best to let yoga chisel away our blind spots and our delusions. We understand that it is an honor and a privilege to be able to study this gift from India, a gift that is science, technology, philosophy, ethics, art, and spiritual practice all rolled into one. We treat the practice with reverence and respect, understanding that we are guests. We seek to understand the roots, history, and meaning of this path, as well as to look critically at the ways it has been appropriated and disrespected.

If you do not yet long for the liberation of all, for the cessation of suffering as well as the well-being, comfort, and peace for all beings, you will. The connection and beauty that can be experienced through your practice will have you yearning for that same connection and beauty to be reflected throughout the world. That yearning will fuel your action, as you will understand deeply that in practicing yoga, you are called to take action, on behalf of others as well as the Earth. The way that life is being lived on this planet, at this time, is deeply unsustainable, unjust, and lacking in basic equality, integrity, kindness, and compassion.

All over the world, people are oppressed, threatened, tortured, maimed, and killed because of their skin color, social status, gender identification, or sexual preference as well as their religious beliefs or tribal affiliation. Perhaps nowhere is this more glaring than in the United States, a stronghold of white supremacy and capitalism. Both of these social institutions are killing the planet, choking the very life out of people and ecosystems. They are so deeply ingrained in everything that they are in fact the water we drink, the air we breathe, the very scaffolding upholding entirety.

Although some practitioners maintain that "yoga is not political," I beg to differ. "Politics" are simply the policies that shape the infrastructure of our lives, and so it seems to me that yoga is inherently political in the sense that it requires a commitment to policies that do not cause harm, policies that do not steal or hoard, policies that are honest and equitable. Furthermore, I would argue that we need to enact policies that recognize the errors and harms of the past and make reparations for the harm done. Because if we don't do this, make meaningful amends for past wrongdoing, then we will never get free. At the heart of many spiritual teachings is the understanding that so long as one of us suffers, none of us are liberated. What is yoga if not (at least in part) a longing for liberation from ignorance and wrongdoing?

If you have never taken political action before, the idea of using your yoga practice to inform your choices and actions in this way might be overwhelming to contemplate. It's okay to feel that, but it's not okay to stay there. My friend Michelle Cassandra Johnson authored an extraordinary book, *Skill in Action: Radicalizing Your Yoga Practice to Create a Just World*. This book was inspired by two verses from the Bhagavad Gita:

> *On this path no effort is wasted, no gain ever reversed, for even a little bit of this practice will shelter you from sorrow.*

> *Yoga is Skill in Action. Do every action to the best of your ability.*

In her book, Michelle observes, "We are living in a space where our lives depend upon our shared humanity in a way that I haven't ever experienced." She goes on to say,

> White supremacy and capitalism are coming for all of us. If we don't begin to consider how our thoughts, words, and actions impact the collective good, we will perish. If we don't begin to work collectively and in solidarity with one another, we will perish. The journey of discovering that our dharma is connected to the greater good is challenging and we must do it anyway. We must skillfully take collective and radical action to create a world that allows all of us to breathe, be, live, be seen, and validated.[*]

In the resources section of this book are suggested books, organizations, and teachers that can educate, inspire, and guide you in your personal actions to create a more just and sustainable world. Take heart and know that this too is part of your practice. And keep in mind that the personal action we must take is not only outside of us but within us as well. When it comes to racial justice and dismantling structures of white supremacy, those of us with power and privilege must be willing to examine the ways in which we have benefited from or caused oppression, ways in which we may have contributed to the harm, knowingly or unknowingly. In the realm of environmental justice, we have to examine our lifestyle and our habits, our appetites and consumption, and pay attention to whether the choices we make are contributing to environmental degradation and climate change or mitigating it. Engaging with our community, our country, and our world with an intention of right action is enormous work, but it's the most important work that we can do.

With our practice itself, do we practice in a studio that offers a diversity of teaching staff? Do the classes we attend or teach reflect the demographics of the community in terms of race, age, and gender identification? Are these classes financially as well as physically accessible to all? Is the studio a place where the practice is respected and the great and universal vows are guiding studio conduct? Or is it a structure of commodification, of prioritizing profit over people, perpetuating harm in numerous ways? Is there an effort to engage the community in deeper study of the roots and teachings of yoga? Does the studio support the community—from offering a gathering place to taking opportunities to serve the surrounding community? These are just some of the questions we should be asking about the places we frequent.

[*] Michelle Cassandra Johnson, *Skill in Action: Radicalizing Your Yoga Practice to Create a Just World* (Radical Transformation Media, 2017), 21.

Ultimately, we not only want to practice in a place that embodies the spirit of yoga, but we also want to perpetuate with intention those places that live the heart of yoga.

Kennae Miller, an inspiring teacher and friend, whose yoga studio serves marginalized and underrepresented communities of Charleston, South Carolina, offered this summation to me:

> To take action in yoga is to be in a practice of noticing what is inactive within us. Noticing what is inactive within us is where we can begin to identify, in our external world, in our communities, and in the world, where we have been inactive. Yoga movement asks us to be in the seat of—whether a posture, withdrawal of the senses, cleanliness, or non-harming. For each of us to do any of these requires us to first take action of noticing and then the action of practicing, yoking the two together. It is then the yoking of taking action and the practice that bring our internal and external worlds together, so we begin to see the world reflected within us and how we are reflected in the world.

I believe, with every fiber of my being, that we all share a knowing. This knowing is deep-rooted and has been with us since we first began to perceive the world as children—possibly this knowing is ancestral. The knowing is that the world does not have to be the way that it is, that a far different world is possible. Together, we understand that this current version is not holding all of us—it is, in fact, harming so many of us. Our relationships with each other, with the natural world, are in extreme disrepair. This is the ache in our hearts. Yoga invites us to sit with that ache, to not turn away but to lean in. That ache has something to say, something to teach. We need only to still ourselves and listen. In listening, the way forward will become clear, the path illuminated a little differently for each of us.

Yoga is a word that has come to represent so very many different things, but recall that it is sourced from the Sanskrit root *yuj*—meaning not only "to yoke" but also "to join," "to unite." And what is a yoke but an implement to join more than one in applying effort to the same goal? Implicit, at the very heart of the practice, is that call: to join, to unite, to yoke with each other in creating "the more beautiful world we know in our hearts is possible."*

---

* The phrase "The more beautiful world we know in our hearts is possible" is the title of a book by Charles Eisenstein. Those words landed in my heart immediately, articulating so simply and so beautifully that ache in the heart, the knowing that we all share.

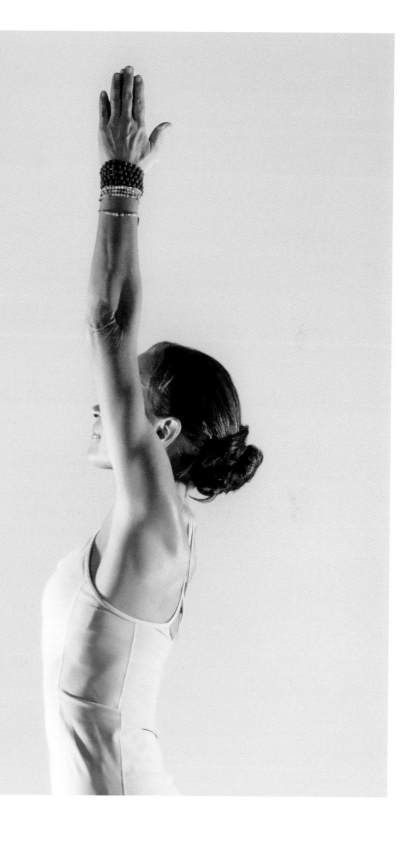

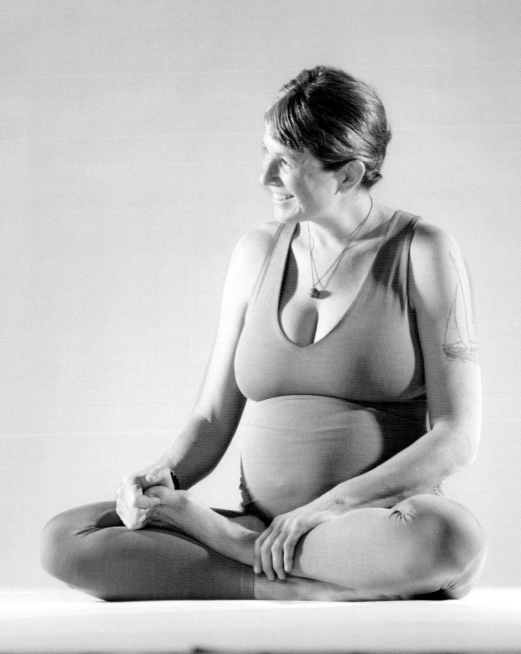

Epilogue

ENCOURAGEMENT

I T HAS BEEN SUCH an incredibly deep pleasure to create *Moon Path Yoga* and to imagine you finding it. To share all that I know about the moon, yoga, and our lunar ways was a dream come true. I fervently hope that *Moon Path* will shape your practice—that you will find these teachings compelling and nourishing. And, however you adopt this offering into your life, it is important to remember, always, that your practice belongs to you. Every single ounce of energy, time, and effort that you put into your practice will forever belong to you and it will live within you. The practice of yoga will teach you and gift you in ways that you can't even imagine right now. Time practicing, on and off the mat, is an investment in your future well-being, your future right action, and your future resilience, while enhancing each moment in the present.

Befriend your body and practice with that friend. Don't worry so much what your practice looks like, nor what you look like. The treasure you seek is truly within you.

When hard times come, and they will and they do, this practice will hold you. Grief, loss, sorrow—they visit all of us, uninvited and unwelcomed, yet what exquisite teachers they are. Carving us right down to the bone, pushing us right to the unfathomable edge of what we can endure, and always, always teaching us.

When joy and comfort, pleasure and ecstasy find us, may they find us with open hands and generosity of heart, willing to share our abundance.

Don't give up. Don't ever give up. Look to the moon and remember that you are not alone. Look to the moon and remember your true and enduring nature. Open the *Moon Path*, choose a practice, and remember your connection and your wisdom. Look to the moon.

Acknowledgments

THIS BOOK IS A SONG of movement and moon, my first and primary languages. I am humbled and grateful to sing it to you. May we feel the beauty of our instinctual wildness and honor our collective hunger for deeper relationship, for respectful, equitable, and sustainable ways of being in community, together on Earth.

We are our ancestors, our families, our friends. No accomplishment is ever achieved alone. I am thankful first, for my mother, Patricia, and my father, William, for giving me life and shaping me. I am the first generation, on my mother's side, to be born in this country and the waters of the lochs, the minerals of the low mountains of Scotland, still thrum in my veins. The salt, rivers, and mountains of Virginia I contain are gifted from my father. I am thankful for my sister Julie for sharing the journey of family with me, and to her husband, Ron, for joining that journey. Zach, Indigo, and Brian are mighty and powerful souls, the loves of my life, my children, and the reason for most everything. Shout-out to Dylan and Jill for being family love too.

My friends are extraordinary; truly I am the richest woman in the world, and this is the wealth that matters. The writing of this book (so lucky to have this opportunity) paradoxically happened during a three-year patch of heartbreak, grief, and challenge. These people kept me going, each, in their own way, a beacon of goodness, of love, of comfort: Heather and Michael, Jen and Scott, Mary and Pete, Amanda and yo fist bump Big Mike, Beth and Steve, Neely, Leslie and David, JP and Leigh, Pete, Mark is love, Michael Johnson, Giuseppe, Poozie and Tom and that whole clan, Michael who is my Michael, Davis who taught me that you can miss someone you haven't met yet, Ethan, Cori, Jesse, Jennifer, Connie, and sweet songbird Chloe. I could keep listing friends for pages but these ones took my breath away.

I will be forever grateful to my editor Beth Frankl for finding and encouraging me, grace and more from Emily Coughlin, and to Shambhala for giving me this opportunity. Annie Killam is not only an amazing photographer who captures beauty wherever she trains her lens, but she is also a dear friend. That too applies to Emily Nicols, arriving to help, hang out, and contribute to the *bhavana*. Gratitude to beloved friend Heather Watrous and her talented daughter Delphi Fishbach for illustrating the moon tracking chart on page 37.

The luminous and beautiful people who illustrate the postures and meditations within are all beloved friends, as well as practitioners of yoga. In order of appearance:

Demacy Kincaid Monte-Parker, myself, Jane Calhelha, Ainhoa Bilbao Cebrero, Byrdi Lee, Indigo Burford, Utah Green, Melody Sufia, Cori Anderson. It occurred to me somewhat belatedly that the models would need clothing. Incredible gratitude to the yoga apparel companies Beyond Yoga and Liquido for generously outfitting the models. Both companies are woman owned and strive for environmental sustainability and ethically sound manufacturing and sourcing as well as utilizing images that represent the beauty and diversity of women's bodies. Deep bow especially to Beyond Yoga for making truly lovely clothing for more voluptuous bodies.

Gratitude to René Roberts and Erin Adams for creating access to their gorgeous studio where the sequences were photographed. Gratitude also to Sue Ann Fisher of West Asheville Yoga, for lending props and bolsters and continually showing up as an all-around kind and beautiful soul. Love, a heart full of love, to my friends and colleagues at Yoga International, for not just offering yoga, but for being yoga.

The love I have for the land I live upon, in the mountains of western North Carolina, is immense. With the utmost respect, I would like to acknowledge that this land belongs to the Anikitugwagi, the Cherokee people. Recognizing this land as Cherokee land is not sufficient to overcome colonialization and Indigenous genocide. I am committed to learning the stories of the original inhabitants of this land, to being in right relationship with and learning from the Cherokee people. I am committed to caring for all the relations of this land and to consider the impacts of my lifestyle on future inhabitants of this land.

The heart and source of much of this book is from the tradition of yoga; the lineages that I draw from originate in South Asia. This area of the world was also subject to brutal colonization and disrespect. The ancient and profound practice of yoga was developed over thousands of years as a path to end suffering, to yoke our disparate aspects of self that we may experience wholeness and, in doing so, apply our life force to the creation of a world where all have access to the experience of wholeness and well-being and none suffer. In direct contradiction to the teachings of yoga, this practice has been appropriated, commodified, objectified, and used for ill gain by many in the Western world. It is a great privilege to be able to practice a revered tradition from another culture. It is my deepest intention and embodied prayer that I share the teachings that my Indian teacher bestowed upon me, with open hands, with respect and accuracy. In the spirit of respect, responsibility, and reciprocity, I honor the obligation of *gurudakshina*, a sacred trust for all who receive the teachings of yoga to repay one's teacher, to repay the origin and source of the teachings.

Resources

PEOPLE

I've referenced some amazing people in this book and here, listed (almost) in the order that they are encountered in the book, are their details.

Shala Worsley is an Ayurvedically influenced yoga teacher, E-RYT 500. She created a National Ayurvedic Medical Association–approved 600-hour Ayurveda Wellness Counselor Certification Program as well as a school for certification in massage therapy and Ayurveda wellness, which she managed for fifteen years. Shala uses the ancient practices of yoga, Ayurveda, and astrology to help groups and individuals navigate modern times with awareness and compassion. Shala is an excellent resource if you would like support in creating personalized programs to balance your doshas. You can reach Shala by emailing her at shala@YogaAndTheCosmos.com.

Vishnu Dass, AD, LMT, NTS, is recognized at the Ayurvedic doctor level of professional membership by the National Ayurvedic Medical Association and has seventeen-plus years of full-time clinical experience. Vishnu created and runs Blue Lotus Ayurveda, an Ayurveda and panchakarma clinic in Asheville, North Carolina. Visit www.bluelotusayurveda.com for more information on services and learning opportunities. Note to the reader: Vishnu was not actually mentioned in the book but was very generous with his knowledge of Ayurveda, and it felt right to list him here.

Thich Nhat Hanh (known as Thay to his students) is a Zen master, global spiritual leader, poet, and peace activist, revered around the world for his teachings on mindfulness, global ethics, peace, and kindness. You can learn more about Thay, his life, his teachings and the many, many books he has written at www.plumvillage.com.

Guru Rattana, PhD, is one of the many teachers whom I have studied with over the years and is especially dear to my heart. She is an author, teacher, and teacher of teachers and has studied kundalini yoga and meditation for forty-plus years. You can learn more about what Guru Rattana has to offer by visiting www.yogatech.com.

Susanna Barkataki is an Indian yoga practitioner in the hatha yoga tradition. The author of *Embrace Yoga's Roots: Courageous Ways to Deepen Your Yoga Practice,* Susanna is a yoga culture advocate and inclusivity promoter. Learn more at www.susannabarkataki.com.

Michelle Cassandra Johnson is a social justice activist, yoga teacher, author, empath, and intuitive healer. Michelle's offerings are extensive, from teacher trainings to workshops to podcasts and books. Learn more at www.michellecjohnson.com.

Kennae Miller is a change invoker, inner work instigator, and yoga teacher. Kennae's studio, Transformation Yoga, is South Carolina's only Black, Veteran, and woman-owned yoga studio. To learn more about Kennae's offerings, visit www.transformationyogasc.com.

BOOKS

I am a reader! I love the experience of traveling and learning through books. Following is an alphabetical ordering of just a few of the books that have been influential for me, specifically with regard to the contents of *Moon Path.*

FUNDAMENTALS

Bhagavad Gita. Numerous translations of this work are available, and I encourage reading the efforts of multiple translators to deepen one's relationship with this text.

Kundalini Tantra. By Swami Satyananda Saraswati. Bogota, Colombia: Yoga Publications Trust, 2007.

The Upanishads. Translated by Eknath Easwaran. Tomales, CA: Nilgiri Press, 2007.

The Yoga Sutras of Patanjali. Numerous translations of this work are available, and I encourage learning from multiple translators to shape one's relationship with the sutras.

ON PRACTICE AND ACTION

Aderin-Pocock, Maggie. *The Book of the Moon.* New York: Abrams Image, 2019.

Barkataki, Susanna. *Embrace Yoga's Roots: Courageous Ways to Deepen Your Yoga Practice.* Orlando, FL: Ignite Yoga and Wellness Institute, 2020.

Gurmukh. *Bountiful, Beautiful, Blissful.* New York: St. Martin's, 2014.

Hanh, Thich Nhat. *How to Love.* Berkeley, CA: Parallax Press, 2015.

Johnson, Michelle Cassandra. *Skill in Action: Radicalizing Your Yoga Practice to Create a Just World.* Portland, OR: Radical Transformation Media, 2017. Reprint, Boulder, CO: Shambhala Publications, 2021.

Khalsa, Nirvair Singh. *The Art, Science and Application of Kundalini Yoga.* N.p.: Kendall Hunt, 2018.

O'Donnell, Kate. *The Everyday Ayurveda Guide to Self-Care.* Boulder, CO: Shambhala Publications, 2020.

Stone, Michael. *Yoga for a World Out of Balance.* Boston: Shambhala Publications, 2009.

Svoboda, Robert E. *Prakriti.* Twin Lakes, WI: Lotus Press, 1998.

Vidal, Mas. *Sun, Moon, and Earth.* Twin Lakes, WI: Lotus Press, 2017.

TRAUMA

I spent some time discussing trauma in chapter 8. Trauma is tricky to unwind and tricky to understand, yet virtually all of us live with some degree of trauma. Further complicating a universal understanding of the nature of trauma is that each of us experiences traumatic events in different ways and we all have different levels of resilience within. Trauma is held somatically, in our tissues and muscles. This is also where we build our levels of resilience: somatically, through connection to friends, family, and practices (for instance, things such as yoga, running, gardening, or art appreciation) that are meaningful and pleasurable. The following books have shaped my understanding of trauma as well as the ways in which we can build our resilience.

Emerson, David, and Elizabeth Hopper. *Overcoming Trauma through Yoga.* Berkeley, CA: North Atlantic Books, 2012.

Levine, Peter A., and Ann Frederick. *Waking the Tiger.* Berkeley, CA: North Atlantic Books, 1997.

Menakem, Resmaa. *My Grandmother's Hands.* Las Vegas, NV: Central Recovery Press, 2017.

Van Der Kolk, Bessel. *The Body Keeps the Score.* New York: Penguin, 2015.

About the Author

SIERRA HOLLISTER seeks to blend her perpetual lovestruck wonder for the natural world with her devoted yoga practice and study. A self-proclaimed "yoga universalist," she is grateful for all traditions and lineages of yoga and the ability to pursue practice as path. In addition to holding teaching certifications in multiple yoga lineages, Sierra is an E-RYT 500 (an Experienced Registered Yoga Teacher with Yoga Alliance) as well as a certified YACEP (Yoga Alliance Continuing Education Provider).

A mother, runner, yoga student, and yoga teacher, Sierra's own yoga journey began with Sarah Powers in 1992. In a beautiful nonlinear way, she was carried to Ahimsa Ashram in Washington, DC. It was here that she fell in love with kundalini yoga, studying with the man who carried the teachings of kundalini from India. Since that time, Sierra has been inspired and shaped by the teachings of many, including Gururattana PhD, Guru Singh, Tias Little, David Swenson, Seane Corn, Pandit Rajmani Tigunait, Kartar Singh, and Michael Stone. The incredibly beautiful souls who have practiced and studied with Sierra over the past three decades have been equally instrumental in teaching Sierra. And while not "yoga," the teachings, writings, and life of Joanna Macy have informed Sierra as much as anything else.

Of all of Sierra's loves, her first and most enduring love was earth, moon, and sun. This love led her to study environmental ethics as an undergraduate and then work at Greenpeace for many years. The natural world continues to beckon her attention, intertwining irresistibly with the great and universal vows of the beginning path of yoga.

Sierra's life, an alchemy of love and yoga unfurls anew each day, perpetually illuminating the obligation to work for social justice, climate justice, ecological justice, and each other. To learn more about Sierra and opportunities to study with her, visit www.sierrahollisterliving.yoga.